stickler

THE ELUSIVE SYNDROME

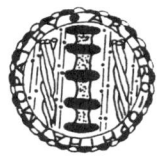

Wendy Hughes

CELTIC CONNECTION

Text © Wendy Hughes 1995

All rights reserved. No part of this publication may be reproduced or transmitted, in any form or by any means, without permission.

ISBN 0 9526625 0 7

Cover design: Susan Skinner
Line illustrations: Christopher Marczewski

Published by:
Celtic Connection
27 Braycourt Avenue,
Walton on Thames,
SURREY KT12 2AZ

Printed in 1995 by Gwasg Carreg Gwalch, Iard yr Orsaf, Llanrwst, Gwynedd, Wales.

DEDICATION

For Tim Weisselberger
who always supplied the inspiration in times of need,
and for all 'Stickler' children past, present and future.

ACKNOWLEDGEMENTS

This book could not have been written without the help, advice and encouragement of many people. I would like to thank everyone who has shared their time and knowledge with me in the production of this book, particularly the medical professionals. Despite very busy schedules, they have painstakingly read my manuscript, listened to my endless questions and supported me in what I have been trying to achieve. Thanks are also due to the affected families who have so generously shared their experiences with me, and who in turn will undoubtedly help other families to cope in a similar situation.

Special thanks to:

Gunnar B Stickler, M.D. Ph.D., Emeritus Staff, Mayo Clinic, Rochester, Minnesota, USA. who answered my first plea for help and put me in touch with numerous families, and has continued to help and encourage me.

Mr R J Cooling, FRCS, FRCOphth, Medical Director, Moorfields Eye Hospital for all his support and encouragement, especially at times of operations. Also his long suffering secretary, Heather Lucas, who has unwittingly become the buffer between us.

Dr Mike Pope, Addenbrookes NHS Trust who helped to unravel the mystery of genetics and enabled me to obtain a reader's ticket for the

Royal Society of Medicine library.

Mr Martin Snead, FRCS, FRCOphth, Senior Registrar, Department of Ophthalmology, Addenbrookes NHS Trust Hospital for his help in understanding recent gene research.

Dr Rai, Senior Registrar, Department of Rheumatology, Coventry and Warwickshire District Hospital for his explanation of joint problems.

Mr D W Patton, Oral and Facial Surgeon, Morriston Hospital NHS Trust, Swansea for his help concerning facial abnormalities, and cleft palate repair.

Dr Karen Temple, Wessex Clinical Genetics Service, Southampton who has always shown a great interest in the book and the Stickler Syndrome Support Group.

All the other professionals and organisations who have so kindly helped, especially Carol Youngs, Assistant Director, Contact-a-Family for her advice and support.

Also thanks to the following:

Jean Sergeant who so freely gave her time to proof-read several versions of the manuscript and for her useful suggestions to improve the readability of the text.

Susan Skinner, who has not only encouraged me in all my writing activities, but designed the cover for this book.

Christopher Marczewski for his amusing line drawings.

Dr Beryl Hazeldine, my History Of Medicine tutor, who introduced me to the wonderful world of medicine, and who has always been willing to obtain information for me, even at a moment's notice.

Molesey Writers Circle for their continuing support, especially Anne Ephgrave who offered help with the chapter concerning genetics.

The Society of Women Writers and Journalists who have always been there when I needed them most.

Stuart McGuiggan, for his fascinating insight into the printing world and helpful advice on producing camera-ready copy and layout.

My husband Conrad who has not only had to put up with me, but has always supported and encouraged, as well as having to live with this book since it's conception.

And last, but certainly not least, my printer, Myrddin ap Dafydd, who has enabled me to see this book through to a satisfactory conclusion. I am sure that there are many more people whom I should have acknowledged but inadvertently forgotten. Thank you and please accept my apologies.

PLEASE NOTE: Although I have little medical knowledge, I have tried, to the best of my ability, to write an accurate account of Stickler syndrome through the eyes of one living and coping with its everyday problems. Any errors or omissions in the text are my responsibility, and I would be extremely grateful for any comments, so that misunderstandings or inaccuracies can be rectified in future editions.

A NOTE ABOUT THIS BOOK

The chapters that deal with specific medical symptoms are divided into two sections. The main body of each chapter outlines the medical side of the condition. The concluding pages consist of a 'Your Questions Answered' section. This is based upon the questions I am frequently asked.

I have, where appropriate, used the medical terms that you will encounter on your visits to the hospital, followed by a simple explanation of their meanings. I have decided to use this format because, being partially sighted myself, I know how frustrating it can be when you are referred to a footnote or a glossary of terms situated away from the main text. It should be possible to identify the terms without having to locate a reference and weave your way back to the correct place in the text. However, I am aware that there will be others reading the book who would prefer a glossary of terms, and for their benefit I have included one at the end.

CONTENTS

Foreword	Gunnar B. Stickler	xiii
Preface	Mr Robert Cooling	xvii
Chapter One	The Quest Begins	21
Chapter Two	Stickler Syndrome and Its Symptoms	39
Chapter Three	Genetics, The Collagen Factor, and The Genetic Implications	67
Chapter Four	The Eyes	91
Chapter Five	The Joints	109
Chapter Six	Oral and Facial Abnormalities	131
Chapter Seven	Other Problems and Worries	151
Chapter Eight	You Are Not Alone and How Others Have Coped	169
Chapter Nine	Coping With A Child Affected By Stickler Syndrome	191
Chapter Ten	Helping Yourself To a Better Way Of Life	205
	Useful Organisations and Addresses	229
	Glossary of Terms	235
	Reading List	238
	List of Medical References	240
	Bibliography	243

FOREWORD

While looking onto the flooded Mississippi from my study, I think about men's continued effort to make order out of chaos. I reflect about the remarkable book Wendy Hughes has written. She describes very well the hereditary disease which we at the Mayo Clinic named 'Hereditary Progressive Arthro-ophthalmopathy'. All the signs and symptoms are listed and clearly explained.

Her own experiences in coping with a hereditary disease must be a great encouragement for the sufferers of this illness. It is society's gain that Wendy's condition was diagnosed and defined. Some order replaced chaos. This alleviated her anxiety about an obscure illness threatening her and allowed her to begin a new career as an author of many articles and a number of books. The topics range from historical essays about her native Wales, the hysterical dancers of Aachen, to among many others, an Austrian physician, Leopold Auenbrugger.

She has much to say about how she and other affected persons have been dealing with their problems. Most impressive is the advice she gives to people on coping with visual difficulties and various joint problems. This book will help not only Stickler sufferers and carers but can help anybody with a chronic illness.

Last but not least, she has founded a much needed Support Group. It is hoped that physicians such as geneticists, ophthalmologists, orthopaedists and others will read this book in order to better understand the condition and how such an illness affects patients.

Gunner B. Stickler
Lake City, Minnesota

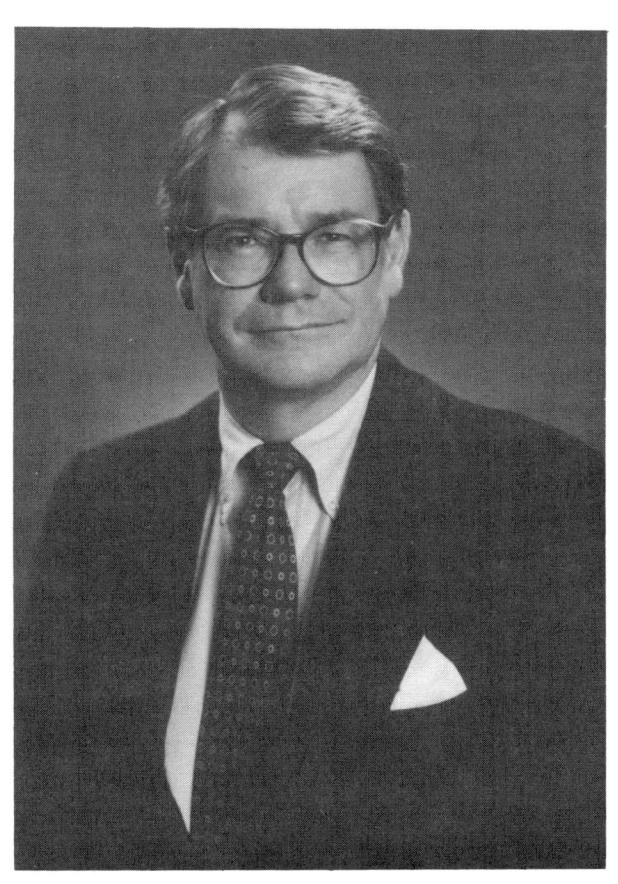

Dr Gunnar B Stickler

PREFACE

It may surprise you to learn that like many doctors I would confess to being once highly sceptical of the idea of patient support groups. This probably stems from the days of my medical training when a little knowledge was always perceived as dangerous. Of course we now live in far more enlightened times when the expectations of patients and their families continue to increase. Understandably there is a wish to participate in the decisions regarding their treatment based upon a better understanding of their conditions. This thirst for knowledge can be difficult and patients who reach for standard textbooks of medicine will often find the information difficult to assimilate and rarely are the concerns and questions in the mind of the lay reader addressed. Similarly, the General Practitioner, the linchpin of the Health Service, may because of a lack of specialist knowledge be unable to advise the sufferer. Patients are often reluctant to ask of the hospital specialist which they fear might seem trite and may be dismissed. All too often, the patient is left feeling isolated and fearful of the worst. As Wendy Hughes taught me, the situation is compounded for the sufferer of an elusive syndrome which can be unfamiliar to many branches of the medical profession.

I must admit that through my dealings with other patients support groups, I have come to appreciate the immense value and benefit to many of my patients who in turn have been able to help others. The opportunities to share a problem can provide more than half of the solution and I never cease to admire the remarkable energy and enthusiasm of those who contribute so much in this way in the support of others.

Ask any doctor who has been in practice for a number of years and they will be able to conjure up a list of their most memorable patients. Inevitably, the list will contain some outstanding treatments, successes or masterful diagnosis as well as miserable and heart-rending failures. There are others who stick in the memory by virtue of their outstanding personality, unique attributes and other remarkable human qualities. It will not surprise you to know that Wendy Hughes is included in my personal list because of her extraordinary spirit, sense of purpose and remarkable courage. Early on in our dealings, it was clear she recognised a job that needed to be done and heaven forbid anyone who stood in her way! The word needed to be spread and who better than Wendy with her talent and zest for the written word to rise to the occasion. The ability to convey the nuts and bolts of a complicated medical condition even for those of us who are medically qualified is an exacting task and is the product of a rare talent which is there to be seen throughout this book.

I feel greatly privileged to be associated with this work and to be asked to provide the introductory remarks. I am in no doubt that from the lucid description of the facets of this disorder and the advice conveyed together with the personal perspective of the author, the reader will gain considerable insight, guidance and assistance in coming to terms with the effects of this chronic ailment. As the author once said to me in a determined voice - 'I'll write about it.'

Robert J Cooling FRCS, FRCOphth
Medical Director &
Consultant Ophthalmic Surgeon
Moorfields Eye Hospital NHS Trust

CHAPTER ONE

MY QUEST BEGINS

Despite various health problems since childhood, it was not until I suffered severe sight difficulties in 1988 that Stickler syndrome was finally diagnosed. My case is typical of many affected by Stickler syndrome who have had years of non-specific illness and no definite diagnosis, yet all the signs and symptoms were there for potential interpretation.

On reflection, I suppose it is easy for me to say this, especially in the light of my own research. Medicine is a huge field and doctors cannot be expected to know about every single disorder. That would be a human impossibility, especially when they are faced with an obscure condition such as this, which has so many different features.

Let me stress that I am in no way laying the blame at the door of the medical profession for the long delay in reaching a diagnosis. Without the expertise of my ophthalmic surgeon, I would not have found a new lease of life or have enough vision to pursue a career in writing. Without the help of my rheumatologist, my joint problems would be less bearable, and without the services of organisations like the Royal National Institute For The Blind, and the local Resource Centre for the visually impaired, life would be a struggle.

The fault, I consider, lies in the lack of awareness of the condition, and I hope this book will in some way help to correct the situation.

Although this is not a book about myself and how I have coped, I feel it is important for me to outline my story because I am sure that those affected will, at one point or another, identify with me. I recently received a letter from a young woman of 21. She wrote that no one would ever know how inadequate she felt at school, being branded lazy and, at times, incapable of comprehending even the simplest of knowledge. My heart went out to her, because I knew exactly how she felt. Until I was diagnosed the feeling of being inadequate and a second rate citizen haunted me.

A young lad wrote saying that he was fed up with continual illness and missing out on school and family outings. He was never chosen for the school rugby or athletics team. The chances of his being unable to attend some big event were too great for the organiser to take the risk of selecting him. Again I can identify with him. Whenever there was something special going on, I was sure to have an infection or joint pain to contend with. I was born and brought up in Wales where it is every little Welsh girl's pride to wear her national costume to school on St. David's Day. My costume, unfortunately, remained in my wardrobe on more St David's Days

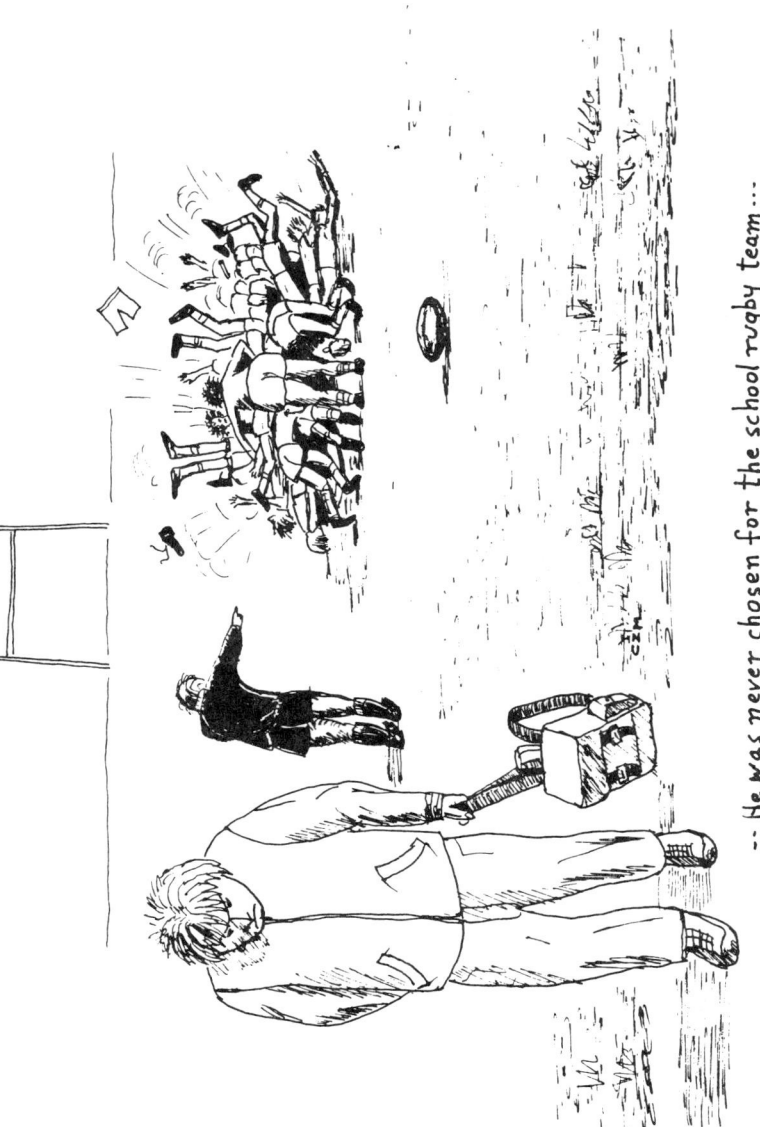

than I care to remember.

Many have written expressing their feeling of guilt at passing on an inherited condition, although most at the time of conception were unaware that they were suffering from Stickler syndrome. Others speak of the responsibility of caring and doing their best for an affected child.

As Stickler syndrome becomes more readily identifiable, future cases will be diagnosed earlier. In the short time since researching this condition I have found evidence of this taking place. It is thanks to numerous doctors, geneticists and community nurses that children are being brought to the attention of the correct medical professionals at an earlier age. This will heighten the chances of them living a near 'normal' life in a world that is still, sadly, geared to the fittest and strongest.

I was born prematurely in 1948 when my mother was 46 years of age. Being her first and only child, I was much wanted but was always 'sickly' and this was put down to my early arrival. It was later discovered that I had been born with a submucous cleft palate and a bifid uvula. In a submucous cleft palate, the lining of the soft palate looks normal, but the deep tissues including the muscles do not join in the midline, so that the palate cannot work properly. This can make feeding very difficult and would try the patience of the most saintly of mothers, as my own can testify. One mother recalls taking up to four hours to bottle-feed her child until she found an answer.

By using a thoroughly sterilised squeezy washing-up bottle with a large holed teat, she could spurt the milk into her baby's mouth and let the droplets trickle down the throat. Thankfully there are now specially designed feeders to cope with this problem. My own cleft palate was never repaired. The only obvious signs are a rather nasal voice, difficulty in pronouncing certain words and a susceptibility to colds, many of them!

Throughout my childhood I ached all over and had difficulty keeping up with other children both academically and physically. Determined to be 'normal' I did my best. Eventually I more or less accepted that I was 'different' from other children, although I didn't understand why.

My mother took me to various consultants. The majority told her she was fussing over nothing. I was born small therefore she could expect a few problems. Usually they said that I was a self-willed little girl who chose to do only the things I wanted to do, and listened only to the things that interested me. I was an attention seeker, a devious manipulator claimed one.

From the day I started school I encountered problems. I was forever ailing with ear infections, caused in part by the cleft palate, although we did not know this at the time. Often my joints would ache and swell up making running and walking difficult. Cold and damp weather affected me greatly and my frequent absence through illness eventually took a toll on my progress at school. Some teachers were understanding and would offer to explain a missed lesson during their breaks, but most were unhelpful, considering me a day-dreamer who was not interested in learning. This could not have been further from the truth. I was extremely interested in all aspects of my education, and still am. But the more I tried to keep up, the more difficult it became.

I was extremely shortsighted and hard of hearing. Even when I sat in the front row in the class, I still had difficulty seeing the blackboard. Having plucked up the courage to ask to sit in the front, I was too shy and nervous to complain again. However, I struggled on and quickly learned the art of copying from my neighbour. Any so-called 'friends' would let me borrow their books to copy up the notes written on the blackboard for the price of a bag of sweets. Despite all the doctors' comments, I certainly wasn't lazy. In fact, in a strange sort of way, I feel that my experiences helped to mould me into the practical, determined person I am today.

My mother had never been a well person, but like many women of her generation, she accepted her lot and got on with life. When I was seven, she suffered severe sight problems, and spent almost a year in and out of hospital. After five failed operations for retinal detachments she returned home totally blind. At the time the detachments were put down to the trauma of my father's sudden death two years earlier.

During this period I was fostered out to a number of families.

One foster mother, being concerned at how close I held a book to my eyes, took me to an optician to have my sight tested. My shortsightedness was discovered and spectacles prescribed. This helped, but I still had difficulties. She also took me to see her GP as she became frustrated at having to call me several times before I would answer, and wondered if I was slightly deaf. The doctors dismissed it as 'attention seeking' on my part, and said it was my way of coping with the absence of my mother. Even today I recall my foster mother's concerns.

From the day my mother returned home, life changed. At the age of eight I grew up rather quickly, when shopping, letter writing, cooking and the 'seeing' things of running a household came under my charge. Her blindness had a profound effect on me. I often closed my eyes to imagine a world of darkness, and would wander around the house refusing to turn on the lights. I would close my eyes and struggle to dress myself, feeling and fumbling for every button. I felt guilty that I could see and my mother couldn't. Often I refused friends' invitations to the cinema and other childhood pursuits. Later, these childhood experiences of trying to appreciate the dilemma of visual impairment helped me to understand my own problems and come to terms with poor vision myself. After all, any vision is better than no vision at all, and I am extremely grateful for what I have.

Home difficulties, coupled with my own health problems, made it increasingly hard for me to keep up with my peers, but I soon found an answer. I would take down the bare bones of the lessons and on my way home from school would pop into the library and find out all I could about that day's lesson. Strangely enough, this fascination with research was to play a major role in helping me to shape a new life later on. I struggled through school and, although I did well considering the problems, it was really because of my extra-mural activities at the library. I even managed to obtain a place at a Technical College for Girls when I was fifteen.

Today my plight might have been quickly recognised and dealt with in a far more sympathetic way. To be fair though, most of my teachers were unaware of the extent of my problems.

After technical college I started work in the buying department of a local engineering firm. Everything was an effort, but I coped well, learning new ways of overcoming old obstacles.

Soon after I began work I met my future husband, Conrad, whom I married two and half years later. He accepted me for what I was and encouraged and supported me in everything I tried to do. For the first time, life was good. There was no need to go on pretending. I no longer had to struggle to keep up with other people. I could simply relax and be myself, and what I found difficult Conrad was only too willing to do.

Our two sons were born within the first four years of our marriage, also a daughter, who sadly died at four months. I relived my own childhood through my children. We would go to see all the

Walt Disney films, visit the zoo, and sit on the swings together. Trips to the sea-side and country-side walks were a pleasure. I enjoyed being a child again - or was it for the first time?

Conrad was a 'new age' modern husband long before the term was invented. We shared the household chores and our sons' upbringing. We did the shopping together, and as I had always found it difficult to do heavy tasks such as housework, bed making etc, he always did more than his fair share without complaint, particularly when I was having yet another bad day. At the time we put this lethargy down to coping with two boisterous youngsters, although deep down I knew there was something wrong. I was different and couldn't understand why I felt like this.

Eventually life began to settle into a contented pattern, the boys were growing up, life wasn't so demanding. Then, when my husband gained promotion in 1980, we moved from Wales to Surrey. The boys were less dependent on me, so I took a part-time job working five mornings a week. For a while this worked and, provided I rested in the afternoon, I coped. In 1984 I made the disastrous decision to take a full-time job. Soon I became extremely tired, my joints became stiff and sore, and I was prone to every infection that came within a two mile radius of me. My vision and hearing seemed to be deteriorating too. I continually put the general ailments down to 'my age'. After all I was now approaching thirty-six, that mid-life stage when parts can be expected to show signs of wear and tear. It is surprising how we can always explain away any problem! A low point was reached during the latter part of 1985 when my joints ached more than usual and I became susceptible to one cold after another. In February 1986 I suffered a viral infection which left me arthritic and lethargic. After about two months of not responding to a variety of antibiotics, my GP referred me to a series of consultants. Tests showed abnormalities, but none could pin-point exactly what was amiss. Most consultants agreed that something was wrong, although one considered my condition to be psycho-somatic. He even suggested that I was becoming paranoid at the thought of my children growing up and preparing to 'flee the nest'. The more I tried to live a 'normal' life, the more incapacitated I became. I began to wonder if it really was 'all in the mind.' Could I be imagining all these aches and pains? Throughout this period my GP was wonderful. He took time to listen to me, and suggested many 'alternative' treatments and relaxation classes, but nothing worked. Finally, a rheumatologist concluded that I was suffering from a post viral chronic fatigue syndrome - sometimes called M.E., and for a while I became more settled. At least someone had given me a label. Although I wasn't fully convinced about this diagnosis, at least someone believed that it wasn't 'all in the mind.'

By now I had been medically retired. As an outlet for my frustrations I turned to my interest in education. To occupy myself I had started to write about incidents in my life, and decided to take this a step further and enrolled for a creative writing course at the local Adult Education centre. This proved most therapeutic because I could 'lose' myself in a piece of writing, and forget the pain I was experiencing. It seemed the mind was willing and able, even if the body had somehow turned into that of a ninety year old woman. I can remember feeling like an inflated balloon with a hole in it. The more I tried to inflate myself, the more I would deflate. I seemed to be running on the spot. By now, Conrad had taken over the organising of the house, all the shopping and washing, besides coping with a demanding full-time job in London.

One day in May 1988, as usual, I had spent the afternoon writing. When I stood up I noticed what appeared to be streaks of black rain falling before my eyes, accompanied by flashes of bright light. For a minute I tried to catch the streaks, thinking it was a cobweb. Perhaps I had done too much close work and was over tired, I thought. Deciding on the latter, I put my work away and made plans for an early night.

The following morning brought little relief, so I went to see my GP. He immediately made an appointment for me to be seen by an ophthalmic surgeon. Within six hours I had been operated on for bilateral retinal detachments. Without the quick actions of my GP, I am sure that I would now be totally blind, and shall always be grateful to him. I know from the many letters I have received that others have not been so lucky.

The operation appeared to go well and after a week I was discharged, but within seven days of returning home the retina in the left eye had detached again. I was rushed back into hospital and was being prepared for another operation when a young doctor came to see me. After a thorough examination of my eyes, he started to ask about my general health, my childhood illnesses, joint problems and my mother's medical history. I can remember being irritated by all these 'unnecessary' questions and wanted to shout, 'I am here for my eyes and nothing else'. Curiously, the prospect of this being a genetic condition had never occurred to me. Finally he put his hand on my shoulder and told me he was cancelling my operation and transferring me to Moorfields Eye Hospital in London. He thought he knew what the problem was, but was not prepared to say anything without a second opinion.

That evening I was transferred to Moorfields Eye Hospital and into the care of Mr Robert Cooling, a surgeon specialising in vitreoretinal disorders. After careful examination and a thorough investigation into my past medical history, he provided me with the reason for all my problems. I was suffering from a common, but little recognised disorder called Stickler syndrome.

I could have hugged him. At last there was a reason for all my difficulties. It was not in the mind after all and, although at this stage I did not understand the implications of Stickler syndrome, I knew this was the key to all my problems. Mr Cooling spoke for about five minutes about the condition, and ended with the words, 'And now you know almost as much about the disorder as I do.' He confirmed that this was also probably my mother's problem. All I could feel that day was immense relief, as though some heavy burden had been lifted from my shoulders. I wanted to shout, 'Look I am not stupid! There's a reason! I am suffering from Stickler syndrome.' It was as though he had given me the final piece to some complicated puzzle. Incidents in my life flashed before me and, for the first time, began to make sense. I cannot put into words the tremendous feeling of relief I felt that day.

The following week Mr Cooling operated on my retina, the first of many operations to save and maintain the vision I have. On the day of the operation, while still heavily bandaged, my husband greeted me with the news that I had sold my very first article to a magazine. These two events signalled a new era for me. From now on I knew that life was going to be good. My life was about to begin.

At this stage I still didn't know what fate held for my vision but after all my earlier struggles I had, through the written word, at last found a way of communicating and I couldn't give up now. All those lovely words that I had been so afraid to say for fear of mispronunciation, were there for me to select at will and use on paper. Unlike speech, it didn't matter if I got it wrong the first time. I could simply cross it out and start again, or shift words around the page at will.

Once home I began to reflect on what Mr Cooling had said about Stickler syndrome. I was convinced that he had not told me everything. I decided that once I was able, I would visit a medical library and find out all about this mysterious condition for myself.

I was appalled to discover that Mr Cooling had been honest and not withheld information from me. Only a limited amount had been written in journals for the medical profession about the condition, and certainly nothing for the lay-person. This, despite Stickler syndrome being considered one of the most common connective tissue disorders. My GP had certainly not heard of it and, as far as I am aware, I am still his only patient with the condition. Intrigued, I wrote to many consultants around the country requesting information. From their replies, it became apparent that some had never heard of the disorder, others knew little more than I did, whilst a few were even amused and thought I had mistaken the diagnosis for Sickle Cell disease - a totally different disorder. One even told me there were only about six affected families in the UK.

However, from the information I collated I learned that in 1965 Dr Gunnar B. Stickler and Associates wrote about a condition called Hereditary Progressive Arthro-ophthalmopathy, now known as 'Stickler syndrome.' The findings were published by the Mayo Foundation, Minnesota, USA, so, frustrated at getting nowhere in my own country, I wrote to the Foundation requesting any information they had.

Much to my delight, I received a reply from Dr Stickler himself, with copies of his report and a follow-up written in 1967. He put me in touch with many sufferers in America, Germany and The Netherlands. My own ophthalmic surgeon passed my name on to affected families in the UK, and correspondence with patients and consultants, both here and abroad, revealed the desperate need for information to avert unnecessary anxiety about the disorder. Hence the birth of the Support Group.

Stickler syndrome affects people in many different ways. Some are so severely handicapped by the condition that life is a continual series of battles. Others are so mildly affected they are unaware they have the condition until a parent or child is diagnosed and investigation reveals that they too have the condition. Between these two bands stand the majority of cases, but most will agree that once Stickler syndrome is diagnosed life becomes more meaningful.

One sufferer described the condition as a 'smorgasbord' of symptoms laid out like a grand feast, without a choice of what is on offer. In this book I have tried to highlight all aspects of the disorder and to be honest without causing alarm. This must always be remembered, because Stickler syndrome is not life-threatening. It can be very inconvenient at times - in fact downright frustrating - but you CAN lead a full and rewarding life if only you allow yourself to do so. This is a condition that is beyond your control, so why not accept the situation and live within your capabilities?

Within my limitations, I achieve far more now than I ever did before it was diagnosed. Knowing what was wrong gave me a wonderful sense of freedom. At last there was no need to struggle to keep up, or feel ashamed of the things I couldn't do. I do what I can, when I can. More importantly, as a direct result of the years of uncertainty, I have discovered my gift of communicating through the written word. I would not have made this discovery, or pursued it without Mr Cooling's diagnosis. Perhaps other sufferers will discover a hidden talent or a new dimension to their lives through diagnosis.

Since that first acceptance in 1988, I have had over 600 articles published. In 1992 my first book was published. This year my seventh book will be published, and two more are due for publication in 1996. Not bad for someone who struggled through school! I have achieved my dream of at last being able to communicate, and if you are determined enough, you too can achieve whatever you wish. The world is your oyster. You and you are alone are in charge of your own destiny.

The main aim of this book is to give sufferers and their families a greater insight into the disorder, and maybe enlighten one or two medical students along the way. Hopefully, I can answer some questions that are of concern, and offer practical advice on the day to day management of the condition. Although I have little medical knowledge, I have tried, to the best of my ability, to explain Stickler syndrome through the eyes of one who is living with it. Only time and research will tell us more. My greatest hope is that my book will inspire someone in the research field to take this disorder seriously, give it the attention it deserves, and provide the necessary funding.

Dr Gunnar Stickler played his part by recognising the problem in 1965, and we must all be thankful for his painstaking dedication. Many consultants in Britain and abroad are fighting their own personal battles to get wider recognition for this condition. I, in a very small way, have tried to contribute by writing this book and setting up the Stickler Syndrome Support Group, which is thriving and continues to grow at an alarming rate. Perhaps, in the not too distant future, all sufferers will be more readily identified and the necessary research undertaken, so that the facts and the best advice and treatments possible are readily available for all affected families.

CHAPTER TWO

STICKLER SYNDROME AND ITS SYMPTOMS

The fact that you are reading this book probably means that you or your family are affected by Stickler syndrome, you care for someone who has the disorder, or are interested to learn more about this common, yet little recognised condition.

If you have been newly diagnosed, then I assume that you know very little about the condition, and feel isolated and frightened about your future. Questions race through your mind and you feel there is no one listening to your queries. Rest assured, you are not alone. These are all very common feelings. The condition is certainly not rare and it is believed that is has been grossly under diagnosed in the past. Stickler syndrome, or ***Hereditary Progressive Arthro-ophthalmopathy,*** is a genetic progressive condition which affects the body's collagen. Collagen is the most plentiful protein in the body - about one third of all our protein is made up of collagen. It forms a major part of connective tissue which can be described as the supportive tissue of the organs of the body in general. Some connective tissue acts like a glue or binding, in other areas it acts like scaffolding, and it can allow for the elastic stretching and tightening, especially in the muscles. Collagen is also an important part of cartilage and bone.

While a baby is being formed in the mother's womb the embryo has a soft cartilage skeleton before the bones are developed. If the wrong collagen units are used, then this may result in faulty shaped bones. In the head this can cause the two halves of the palate not to fuse together, causing a cleft palate, a flat face with a small jaw, a small nose and little or no nasal bridge. Collagen is also found in the cartilage, which covers the bone ends of joints. In the eye it is found in the sclera, cornea and vitreous humour. Therefore these are the areas in which those affected can expect problems.

Recent research has shown that a defective gene called COL2A1 which codes for type 11 procollagen, and is found on chromosome 12, is a possible cause of Stickler syndrome in some families. Other defective genes may be in COL5A1 and COL11A1, and investigations are continuing. The genetic side of the condition will be discussed and explained more fully in Chapter Three.

Stickler syndrome is unusual as there is a great variation in symptoms, even within a family, and this can lead to difficulties in diagnosis, as many families have found. Although the list of symptoms is long there is only a slim chance that a patient will suffer from every feature. The severity of each symptom can also range from not knowing you have a problem, to a slight awareness of a

FAMILY TREE

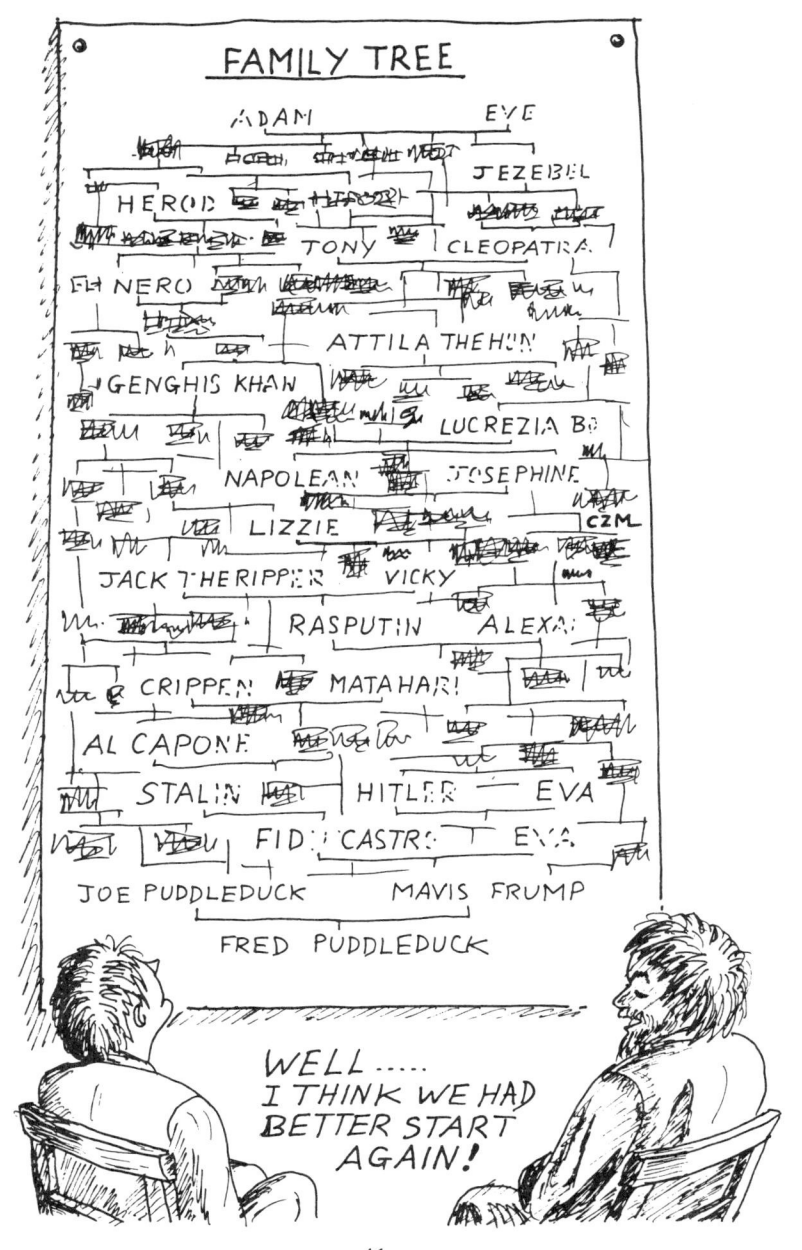

ADAM — EVE
...
JEZEBEL
HEROD
TONY — CLEOPATRA
NERO
ATTILA THE HUN
GENGHIS KHAN
LUCREZIA B.
NAPOLEAN — JOSEPHINE
LIZZIE
JACK THE RIPPER — VICKY
RASPUTIN — ALEXA
CRIPPEN — MATA HARI
AL CAPONE
STALIN — HITLER — EVA
FIDEL CASTRO — EVA
JOE PUDDLEDUCK — MAVIS FRUMP
FRED PUDDLEDUCK

WELL..... I THINK WE HAD BETTER START AGAIN!

difficulty, through to a severe impairment that requires the patience and expertise of a consultant specialising in the relevant field of medicine.

Each case *must* be assessed by a doctor who understands the patients condition, like a geneticist or an ophthalmologist with an interest, and those affected should never assume the worst without discussing problems with those who know more, although on the other hand, don't be too disappointed if you are told that the prognosis (future outlook) is uncertain. No one can foretell how or if a condition might develop.

Absolute truthfulness and acceptance of the situation are the most important factors in coming to terms with the disorder. Any worries should be discussed immediately with your GP or consultant. Often, there is a simple explanation to a query, and a lot of anxiety can be alleviated by seeking advice early.

Only when Stickler syndrome has been properly diagnosed can the genetic implications be made clear to the patient and the family. Other close members of the family may want to be assessed and, where possible, a family tree drawn up, preferably with the assistance of a geneticist. Any connected medical problem can then be uncovered, assessed and the correct treatment undertaken.

The clinical findings can be divided roughly into three groups - eyes, joints and facial appearance. Signs from one group can be greater than another. Also the pattern of symptoms or severity of those symptoms cannot be presumed from previously affected relatives.

MAIN SYMPTOMS

EYES

Myopia (shortsightedness or nearsightedness) - Myopia is generally severe (minus 8 dioptres or more) and evident from birth, but it has also been shown to remain stable over many years. The most harmful symptom of Stickler syndrome is progressive myopia, which in turn, increases the chances of retinal detachment. In 40% of cases, myopia develops before the age of ten and in 75% of cases by the age of 20.

Vitreoretinal degeneration - This means that the small space lying behind the iris and the lens, called the vitreous chamber, is imperfect. The area is normally filled with a jelly-like substance called vitreous humour. In people affected by Stickler syndrome this jelly is improperly formed and is mostly liquid, producing floating, whitish, translucent lines.

Tears and breaks in the retina - These are holes and tears that occur in the inner lining of the eye. They are frequently large, multiple or both and can recur at any time. Generally the retinas in a person affected by Stickler syndrome are in a poor condition, and many surgeons talk of the retina as having a 'lacy' appearance.

Retinal detachments - A detachment occurs when the retina and the underlying inner wall of the eye part company - like wallpaper peeling off a wall. When this happens the peeled off part of the retina will not work properly and the picture that the brain receives becomes patchy or, in some cases, may be completely lost. Detachments can be corrected surgically *if* recognised and dealt with early, although they can be very difficult to repair. Regular checks must be followed up to detect any early detachments. Therefore, the sooner they are diagnosed and operated on, the better the chance of saving useful sight. Early diagnosis is *vital* if blindness is to be prevented.

Early cataracts - This is the clouding or opacity of the lens located inside the eye. This affects the passage of light-rays through to the retina. Although this is a very common finding in Stickler patients, once the cataracts have been removed there is the consolation that the cataracts will not recur.

Secondary glaucoma - This is a condition where the pressure in the eye increases. Left untreated it can lead to visual impairment. In this disorder obstruction of the normal circulation and outflow of the aqueous humour occurs, causing the pressure to rise with irreversible damage to the optic nerve.

BONES AND JOINTS

Premature degenerative joint disease - large bony joints with early onset of degenerative arthritis. There can be a high degree of stiffness or an abnormal amount of flexibility in the joints. The joints mainly affected are the ankles, wrists and knees. Sometimes there is also reduced tension in the muscles. Symptoms are variable and age dependent, and often so mild that only X-rays reveal that changes are present.

Scoliosis - curvature of the spine.

Kyphosis - hump back or angular deformity of the spine.

Genu valgum - The knees are bent inwards - knock kneed.

Coxa valga - deformity of the hip joint in which the angle made by the neck and shaft of the femur is greater than normal.

FACIAL AND ORAL FEATURES

Pierre-Robin Sequence - This is a group of findings which can include a cleft palate or other palatal abnormalities, a small jaw, and a tongue which is relatively too long for the mouth.

Malocclusion - This is poor contact between the chewing surfaces of the upper and lower teeth. Regular dental visits are essential and the expertise of an orthodontist may be required.

Cleft palate - This is a groove or a split in the midline of the palate, caused by the two sides failing to fuse when the embryo is still developing in the womb. This can also take the form of a bifid uvula, submucous cleft palate or a high arched palate. Sometimes only part of the palate is affected or the split may extend for its whole length, with two splits in the front of the maxilla (the upper jaw). It may also be accompanied by a harelip, although this is extremely rare. These conditions can interfere with the formation of the teeth causing overcrowding of teeth.

Hearing loss - This is usually sensorineural, a condition that affects the sensory nerves, but may be caused by otitis media or glue ear. Otitis media occurs when the tube linking the middle-ear to the back of the nose becomes blocked and a jelly-like fluid, naturally secreted by the ear, becomes thicker, filling the middle ear cavity and reducing hearing to a muffled roar.

Facial characteristics - A flat facial profile which can be accompanied by a small button nose and little or no nasal bridge.

Mandibular hypoplasia - a condition where the lower jaw is underdeveloped.

Maxillary hypoplasia - a small upper jaw.

Appearances tend to become less pronounced with age.

OTHER CONDITIONS WHICH MAY OCCUR INCLUDE:

Learning difficulties - Stickler syndrome can present with a variety of learning problems, which can be worrying for a parent. This is not because the child is in any way mentally subnormal - this is *NOT* a symptom of Stickler syndrome. It is caused by poor hearing and sight which slows down development. However, a child diagnosed early will be monitored carefully and the correct educational assistance offered. Progress may also be delayed because lessons are missed due to illnesses, hospital appointments and operations, or because of difficulties in getting about (especially in winter when joints are stiff and swollen). In severe cases the services of a home tutor should be considered.

Stature - Height is generally normal, but some Stickler syndrome patients suffer from a condition where the long slender bones of the hands and feet are abnormally long. This has often led to a mistaken diagnosis of Marfan syndrome, which is also a connective tissue disorder. Other sufferers, however, are short in stature, particularly where there is a history of the condition in several generations.

Mitral valve prolapse - a condition where a valve in the heart fails to close properly and allows blood from the left ventricle to flow back into the atrium. This is a common condition in the general population, but is probably more common in people with Stickler syndrome.

WHY STICKLER SYNDROME?

Stickler syndrome takes its name from the man who first recognised and reported the condition. Gunnar B. Stickler was born in Peterskirchen, a small Bavarian town, on 13th June 1925. He was educated at the Wilhelmsgymnasium in Munich and trained in medicine at the Universities of Vienna, Erlangen and Munich, where he graduated in 1949. Two years later he emigrated to the USA and served an internship at the Mountainside Hospital in New Jersey, and became a resident consultant in pediatrics at the Mayo Clinic.

He obtained a Ph.D at the University of Minnesota. Then, after serving for one year at the Roswell Park Memorial Institute as senior cancer research scientist, he rejoined the Mayo Clinic staff in 1957. From 1959 to 1980 he was Professor of Pediatrics, and chaired the Department of Pediatrics, which at that time had become part of the Mayo Medical School.

He was visiting professor in many institutions in the USA, Austria, Belgium, France, Germany, Iran, Italy, Japan, Sweden and the United Kingdom. He is a member of the American Board of Pediatrics, as well as many other societies and academic committees. He has published over 200 articles on a wide range of paediatric topics, and has served on the editorial boards of clinical journals such as *Clinical Pediatrics, The European Journal of Pediatrics* and *Pediatrics*.

In 1989 Dr Stickler retired from active practice and now enjoys sailing, cross-country skiing and is an ardent iceboater. He lives in Lake City, Minnesota on the shores of Lake Pepin, a natural lake of the Mississippi. He is married, has a son and daughter, and recently joined the realms of grand parenthood, which he enjoys very much.

Gunnar Stickler's quest into Stickler syndrome began back in 1960, when he examined a six-year-old boy at a 'Crippled Children's Clinic'. This was a free clinic staffed by Mayo Clinic physicians. The child had bony enlargements of several joints and was extremely short-sighted. His mother was totally blind, and also had joint problems. Through general conversation, Dr Stickler discovered that many members of this family had similar problems. At one time or another they had all been treated at the Mayo Clinic, the first being examined by Dr Charles Mayo in 1897.

This prompted Dr Stickler to study the family in detail. He was convinced that, in some way, their problems were connected. For the next five years he and his colleagues worked together in an effort to define this disease.

The results of this study formed the basis of their report, which was published in June 1965, in the *Mayo Clinic Proceedings*. Using information collected from five generations of this family, Dr Arthur C. Steinberg MA provided the genetic analysis. It soon became obvious from his research that the syndrome - meaning a collection of signs and symptoms - is caused by an autosomal dominant gene. All genes come in pairs, and by dominant we mean that only one copy of the pair of genes causing Stickler syndrome needs to carry the mutation, or change, for the condition to be present. Autosome genes are found on chromosomes, and there are 23 pairs. One pair are the sex chromosomes and the others are called autosomes and are labelled numerically. It was also noted that the severity, or the variable expression of the condition, can be extremely wide, even within an affected family. These variations in expressivity and severity are typical of disease transmitted by an autosomal dominant gene.

Dr Stickler tentatively named these findings, *Hereditary Progressive Arthro-Ophthalmopathy*. The other authors of that report renamed the condition Stickler syndrome.

The most important discoveries, however, were those relating to ailments of the eyes. A major symptom was severe shortsightedness (nearsightedness), often associated with degenerative changes and sometimes total retinal detachments that can occur suddenly for no apparent reason. It was also found that eyes in which the retina had become detached later developed secondary glaucoma. Complicated cataracts and chronic inflammation were frequently present too. Sadly, in some cases secondary glaucoma went unnoticed, and it eventually became necessary to remove the eye in order to alleviate the severe pain experienced by the patient, and which is caused by the sudden or prolonged rise in pressure.

The joint appearances were studied in detail and the wrists, elbows and ankles were found to be the most affected. Less common were the effects on the joints of the shoulders, spinal column and fingers. X-rays showed that there was a gradual progression of deterioration from the first decade of life onwards.

It was also noted from a genetic point of view that three members of this family had a cleft palate. At the time Dr Stickler did not place any importance on this finding.

Even with so few case histories to study, those early findings showed that the condition varied greatly. For example, a woman born in 1862 had lost all vision in her right eye at the age of eight. A cataract was noted at the age of 12 and bleeding into the eye occurred at the age of 15. At 37, in 1899, her vision had deteriorated so much in the left eye that she was unable to read. When she was examined at the Mayo Clinic in 1907 the eye was painful and protruding. Dr Mayo performed an iridotomy - an operation on the eye in which a hole incision is created in the iris to release the pressure. When she was re-examined in 1913, she was found to have only faint light perception and the lens was opaque. The patient, who lived until she was 68 was known also to have 'large ankles', to walk sideways on her feet and suffer severe pain in her ankles and knees.

Another woman highlighted in the same report was obviously not so badly affected. She was born in 1932, and had progressive myopia which started when she was between nine and 12 years of age. She did not complain of painful joints, although she did experience pain in her ankles if she walked for a long distance. This symptom may well have been an early indication of joint involvement.

From my own research I have found that the condition affects people in many different ways. One young man is very severely handicapped by the condition. His vision is badly impaired, he is profoundly deaf, and has recently undergone a series of operations for severe joint problems. Yet, despite all these problems he is still a 'normal', mischievous boy. His mother told me that recently she needed to shout at him for being naughty. With a large grin on his face he put his two hands up to his hearing aids and switched them off, saying that he could not hear her. Before transferring to a senior school, he attended an ordinary junior school but had difficulty walking. So with the aid of a child seat on the back of her bike, his mother cycled the mile or so to school with him in tow, until she became concerned for their safety. One day he discovered where the brake was located and whenever they reached a crossroad, he stretched out his foot and braked hard.

Another sufferer is so slightly affected that she is aiming for a black belt in karate. Another who has been totally blind in one eye from the age of six is studying A Level art and is hoping to train as an art therapist. She does almost everything that you would expect a '90s' teenager to do, although disco dancing and contact sports are prohibited because of the fragile state of her remaining retina. She studies with the aid of talking books, magnifiers and a word processor which has a magnifying facility. Another two teenagers are hoping to gain the appropriate grades to enter university this year. Really, there is very little a person affected by Stickler syndrome cannot do. It is just a matter of finding the best way to overcome obstacles.

In 1967 Stickler carried out a further investigation of six members of the original family studied. The X-ray films showed many irregularities of the vertebral bones in the chest and lumbar regions. Audiograms recorded on the little boy and his mother some ten months later, revealed that a hearing loss had occurred.

In 1971, Dr John Opitz addressed the American Academy of Ophthalmologists (consultants specialising in eye disorders) and Otolaryngologists (consultants specialising in hearing disorders) and made a strong appeal for further studies into the condition. He also suggested that ophthalmologists examine the face and mouth areas for other defects. He concluded his address by stressing that it was the responsibility of ophthalmologists and their colleagues to educate and co-operate with each other to identify this condition in patients.

In 1972, Opitz and colleagues made another urgent appeal, this time in the *New England Journal Of Medicine*, for the early diagnosis and treatment of patients with Stickler syndrome. They hoped that the genetic implications could be highlighted to affected families, and that more awareness of the condition might prevent blindness. Dr Opitz concluded by saying that it appeared that Stickler syndrome was the most common autosomal connective tissue disorder in the North American MidWest, where he had undertaken his research. Dr Opitz also felt that it is such a common disorder that there are literally thousands, both in the UK and the USA, who are walking around totally unaware they have the condition.

In 1973, Dr Schreiner and colleagues also made a similar appeal and they recommended X-raying all patients with the Pierre-Robin sequence to establish whether they were in fact suffering from Stickler Syndrome.

In 1974, Gillian Turner writing in the *Australian Paediatric*

Journal, reported on a family with the Pierre-Robin sequence and severe myopia. She too emphasised the need for early diagnosis and genetic counselling. In the case she studied, the mother of the family was totally blind and mildly mentally retarded, although her mental state was not associated with Stickler syndrome. She had produced ten children - five of whom were abnormal. Three had died in infancy and two were placed in institutions when the parents could no longer care for them. Gillian Turner pointed out that this woman had not received genetic counselling during any of her ten pregnancies, even though she and five of her children were born with cleft palates. She suggested that genetic counselling and family planning services should be made available as a matter of urgency in all major maternity hospitals.

Another study carried out in 1974 by two Canadian doctors, James Popkin and Robert Polomeno, reported on 22 members of two families who were known to have Stickler syndrome. The most interesting of these findings, published in the *Canadian Medical Association Journal*, were the results of urine samples. Six patients, known to have Stickler syndrome, showed an abnormally high urinary hydroxyproline level - amino acids found only in collagen. The doctors believe an increased level of hydroxyproline may prove useful in diagnosing Stickler syndrome.

In 1975, a Dr Herrmann drew attention to the many separate symptoms of Stickler syndrome which may alert a patient to seek medical advice. He pointed out that where severe myopia, evidence of a cleft palate or unexplained juvenile joint involvement and general non-specific aches and pains were present, Stickler syndrome should be considered. He also estimated that about half of all patients with the Pierre-Robin sequence may also have Stickler syndrome. In addition, since cardiac defects are frequently associated with the Pierre-Robin sequence, he felt that congenital heart disease may also be a symptom of the Stickler syndrome. He and his colleagues also pointed out that the infant mortality rate in Stickler families was high. In Dr Stickler's study evidence was found of two stillbirths and three early deaths. Opitz reported one stillbirth in his 1972 report and Schreiner's 1973 report detailed one stillbirth and one early death. Gillian Turner also reported three early deaths in the family she studied. Again, many families have told me about stillbirths or unexplained infant deaths, even though Stickler syndrome had not yet been diagnosed. Thankfully, with the advent of special care baby units, these problems are dealt with from the moment of birth, giving babies a far better chance of survival.

It is interesting to note that on one particular day at a cleft palate clinic in Great Fall, Montana, Dr John Opitz reported that half of the children seen were later diagnosed as suffering from Stickler syndrome. He is now working on the basis that every child with a cleft palate examined at the clinic is a potential Stickler syndrome sufferer.

YOUR GENERAL QUESTIONS ON STICKLER SYNDROME ANSWERED

I have just been diagnosed and feel so alone. Do others feel the same?

Almost every person I contact with the condition says that once they were diagnosed they felt lost, bewildered and isolated. They did not know where or who to turn to for help and support. Seven years ago I experienced the same worries. The medical profession are usually sympathetic to your plight, but often they cannot tell those affected much about the condition, its prognosis, or how best to cope with the day to day management of organising their lives.

Most who are affected told me that, once over the initial shock of diagnosis, they went through a sort of numbness before they could eventually come to terms with the condition - almost like a bereavement. Some took on a couldn't care less attitude, becoming brash and arrogant, whilst others, like myself, speak of feeling total relief after years of being misunderstood, misjudged and misdiagnosed. All these reactions are quite normal and are part of the 'healing' process. It is important at this stage to talk to others living with the condition. The Stickler Syndrome Support Group offers support, and will put newly diagnosed families in touch with others who are in their own area or experiencing similar difficulties. Also, finding out as much as you can about the disorder helps. It is only when you have all the facts before you that you can assess the situation and begin to put your life together into some sort of order.

How many people are affected by Stickler Syndrome?

According to the Center for Birth Defects Information Services in USA, it is estimated that 1 in every 20,000 people suffer from Stickler syndrome, about 5,000 of the UK population. However, in his book *'Arthritis and Allied Conditions'* - a textbook of Rheumatology - R. E. Pyertiz estimates that the occurrence is as high as 1 in 10,000, and further research may prove the correct figure is much higher, possibly as high as 3 in 10,000 according to some geneticists. Stickler syndrome is far more common than textbooks would lead us to believe. Membership of the Stickler Syndrome Support Group proves this and a recent radio broadcast on the disorder yielded over 100 enquiries from families, Gps, community nurses and rehabilitation officers, proving that a lack of awareness seems to be the key problem.

What is the cause of Stickler Syndrome?

It is still not certain, but there is evidence that Stickler syndrome is caused by a fault in a type of collagen, which is a major protein to be found in vitreous humour and cartilage. This is explained in detail in Chapter Three.

Can Stickler Syndrome be detected at birth?
It can be detected at birth where the Pierre-Robin sequence is present, or where there is a known family history. In most cases, though, it is not diagnosed until mid-life, or until another member of the family is diagnosed. Therefore once one member of a family has been diagnosed it is important for other members to seek medical advice too.

Can I do anything to prevent Stickler Syndrome?
As yet, there is no known prevention, or way of telling if a child will be affected, or, if affected, how mild or severe the results will be. Again, anyone with a family history of the disorder, especially those who intend to have children, should seek genetic counselling.

Is it a life-threatening condition?
It is not a life-threatening condition, and the life span is usually normal. The Stickler Syndrome Support Group's oldest member is 92, and although she has been totally blind and arthritic for over 40 years, she continues to enjoy life within her limitations.

If my child is affected, what are his or her future prospects?
Thanks to more awareness about the disorder the future looks much brighter. It is most important that you treat a child affected by Stickler syndrome as you would any other child.

If Stickler syndrome is diagnosed at, or shortly after, birth special management of the problems of a short jaw and a cleft palate will take priority to enable the child to feed and thrive properly.

Later a speech therapist is important for speech development, and hearing and sight difficulties should be carefully monitored, so that they can be detected early, and the child given the best educational opportunities. It must also be remembered that visual disability exists in a majority of cases from the age of 10 or before, and joint mobility can be a problem throughout life. Later a choice of career should be discussed with those monitoring a child's medical care.

How does an adult cope, when in mid-life they are suddenly told they have Stickler Syndrome?

Most come to terms with the situation easily, because, once over the initial shock, they suddenly find they have the answers to many unexplained problems.

Once Stickler syndrome is diagnosed in the older person, acceptance of living with a progressive condition has to be considered. The avoidance of all exertion, including contact sports, should be carefully observed to preserve the retinas and unnecessary wear and tear on joints. The sufferer should also be encouraged to take up an absorbing interest or hobby that will not aggravate his or her condition. This is *vital* for the patient's well-being and morale, and helps one to feel in control of life once more. With a little adaption there is plenty to do.

I have so many worries and questions to discuss with my doctor. How can I best deal with this?

First work out exactly what is worrying you. Then take each problem separately and ask yourself if your fears are justified. Always divide your anxieties into manageable questions and deal with one at a time. Write them down on paper if it helps. Discuss your problems with the people closest to you. If you are still worried, seek advice from a trained professional dealing with your case. Make an appointment with your doctor and tell the receptionist that you have several questions to ask your doctor. She can then decide whether to book you in for a longer appointment or give you the last appointment of the session, so that neither you nor your doctor will feel hurried. When you arrive say that you have a few questions to ask. Don't rush, and refer to your piece of paper if necessary. Write down any important points discussed, as it is so easy to forget. Never be afraid to ask a consultant what he means. Doctors are used to using certain medical words and forget that many are a mystery to us. Never suffer in silence.

I have heard that people who are affected by Stickler Syndrome become tired easily. If this happens to me, how can I deal with this?

Most people affected by Stickler syndrome, especially children, become extremely tired very easily. This is because the effort of coping with a progressive disorder saps up energy. Pain is also energy destroying. However, this need not be a problem if you learn to pace yourself. There is no need to impose rest on yourself or a child, but be aware of the need to cope within your limitations. A

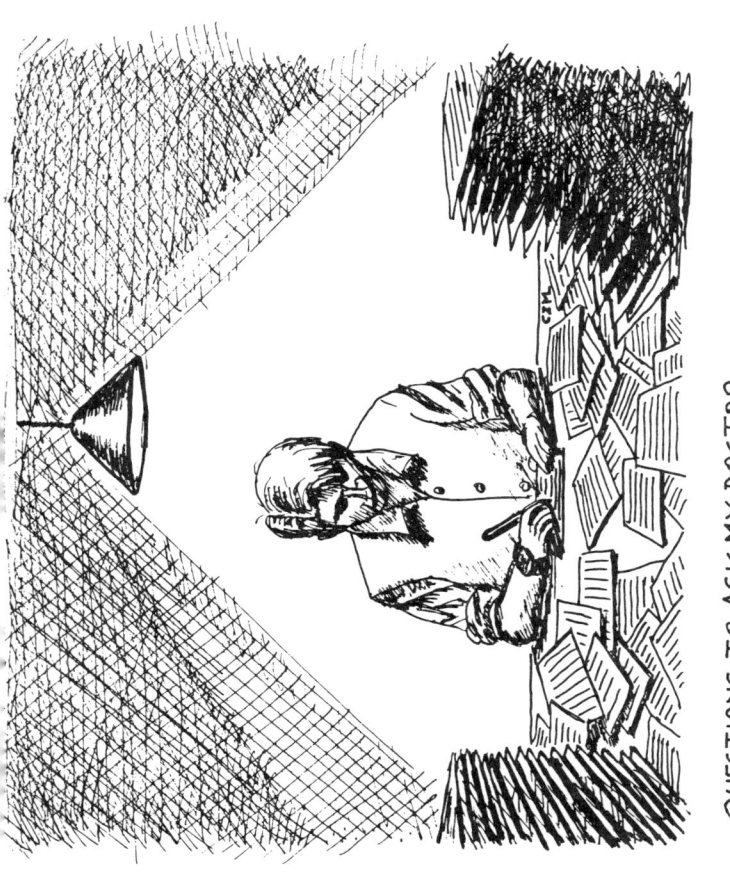

QUESTIONS TO ASK MY DOCTOR......
Write them down on paper

short 10-minute break, when you are beginning to feel tired, can make the difference between a happy relaxed day instead of one spent in misery owing to over-tiredness resulting from pushing yourself too far. When out shopping always make a point of stopping for a coffee break half way through the session.

Muscle weakness can also present problems when simple tasks like bed-making and carrying shopping become exhausting. For some ladies even the weight of carrying a handbag can be a problem, but this can be rectified by carrying a shoulder bag over the shoulder and across the body - thus distributing the weight. Reading a tabloid newspaper can be arduous too, and the affected person may find it more comfortable to read at a table, resting the elbows on the surface of the table so that weak arm muscles are supported. The secret is to identify the difficulty and find an easy way to cope with it.

Remember the old advice: *Never stand when you can sit*. Most household jobs, like peeling potatoes, ironing and rolling out pastry, can be tackled in the sitting position, and will relieve aching joints. Be kind to yourself. There is always an answer to any difficulty if you take the time to think through the problem.

I know from bitter experience that tiredness has no respect for its victims and can strike at any inconvenient moment. It can occur in the middle of a social engagement, whilst visiting, sitting on a train or even out shopping. Often I have become so tired when shopping or visiting that I have to find a quiet corner to have a 'cat-nap' for 5-

10 minutes to enable me to muster enough energy to make the return journey. If you know you are going to do something active or go somewhere special, the key to coping is to rest beforehand and pace yourself during the event. Sit whenever possible and don't be afraid to tell friends you may have to leave early or need extra rests during the day. I know from experience I cannot do two things in one day. If I have an evening event planned, then I don't shop or visit friends during the day. I find I tend to have more energy in the morning, so if I need to go shopping or do anything strenuous I always plan to do these tasks in the morning. It is simply a case of being in control, being sensible and having some respect for your condition. If you are planning to move house, perhaps you should consider finding a home close to your place of work to avoid over-fatigue. Always make life easy for yourself. You would not abuse your car, so do not abuse your body.

How do I cope with tiredness in a child?

The problem of tiredness is frustrating enough for an adult, but is even more difficult for a young child to understand. How do you explain to them why they are suddenly overcome by tiredness, especially when their friends are playing football, swimming or chasing each other around the garden? Without making a fuss, I feel it is important to be completely honest with a child about the condition.

Try channelling their interests into a less stressful hobby or sport, or perhaps suggest to a boy that he could help his football team by becoming their team manager. If children grow up knowing they are a little 'special', then they should be able to cope better. Most children appear to have an inner ability to cope with their prevailing condition.

My teenager, affected by Stickler Syndrome, is becoming difficult. Is there any help available for youngsters?

Teenagers and young adults may need supportive counselling, especially as they reach puberty. They have many questions that they feel they cannot discuss with a parent. Most genetic centres can be of assistance in finding the appropriate person to contact. The Stickler Syndrome Support Group has a Youngsters Network and many have found it beneficial to talk to another affected person of a similar age who has the disorder. This has proved most beneficial where surgery has been recommended and the young person can speak to someone who has had the same or a similar surgical procedure, although it must be remembered that Stickler syndrome varies considerably from person to person even within the same family.

Which doctors need to be involved?

With most rare disorders, GPs know little about the condition, and will need to enlist the services of a number of specialists. In the early days these may include a Special Baby Care Unit and paediatrician. Most diagnosed patients will require help from an ophthalmologist, audiologist and rheumatologist and maybe a social worker and a speech therapist.

It is also important to have one person who understands Stickler syndrome and can offer advice on prognosis, inheritance traits, possible help and treatments available. Most medical geneticists fulfil this need, and the address of your nearest centre can be obtained from the Genetic Interest Group. Address under *Useful Organisations and Addresses*. If you are registered partially sighted or technically blind the services of a rehabilitation officer are invaluable. Regular checks by an ophthalmic surgeon for early detection of retinal detachment, management of cataracts and exclusion of glaucoma are *essential*. Make sure you keep all ophthalmic appointments, and be aware of any changes in vision, particularly in children.

Do all people affected by Stickler Syndrome have a cleft palate?

The majority of those affected with Stickler syndrome have a cleft palate, or some mild abnormality of the palate formation. Many tell stories of feeding difficulties in the past, but thankfully there are various aids and techniques to help. See Chapter Six.

How can I help detect a visual loss in my child?

Tragically, children often accept loss of sight in one eye and say nothing. If you suspect a problem, or a change in vision, however insignificant you may feel it is, consult your GP or ophthalmic consultant immediately.

Is there anything I can do to help detect vision changes early?

Yes. The Stickler Syndrome Support Group has produced an excellent booklet, written by a parent of a child affected by Stickler syndrome entitled 'Care of a Child with Stickler Syndrome.' A copy of this can be obtained from the Group for the price of an A5 stamped addressed envelope.

Can I live a 'normal' life once Stickler Syndrome is diagnosed?

Yes. A full and rewarding life can be lived, *provided* that you accept your situation and live within your capabilities.. You will never feel 100% fit, but then, neither does any able-bodied person. Most who are affected agree that once a diagnosis has been reached and the disorder fully explained, life becomes more meaningful. You may at some stage have to consider a career change, but most importantly, a positive attitude will enhance your outlook on life.

I have heard various other syndromes linked to Stickler Syndrome. Does this mean I have more than one disorder?

A number of doctors have described other conditions in families with similar symptoms to those of Stickler syndrome, and this has caused considerable confusion as to whether these condition are the same or different. These include Marshall syndrome, Weissenbacher-Zweymuller's syndrome or Wagner syndrome. In the past there was much debate within the medical profession as to whether these syndromes were part of Stickler syndrome or not. It now seems likely that as research into the errors in the Stickler gene takes place with more families, this dispute will be resolved once and for all.

CHAPTER THREE

GENETICS, THE COLLAGEN FACTOR AND THE GENETIC IMPLICATIONS

As we have already established, Stickler syndrome is a condition that is caused by what is known as a faulty autosomal dominant gene. Therefore the whole field of genetics, the study of inheritance and heredity, is of interest to a Stickler patient. Genetic research is very much in the news these days and advancing every day, but its study is not a new idea.

From Chaldean engravings produced over 6000 years ago, we learn that even then man was intrigued by inheritance. From these early drawings we can see that these cave dwellers portrayed the inheritance of certain characteristics found in the manes of families of horses.

In 1814 Joseph Adam, an apothecary-physician who lived in London, published a book entitled *a Treatise On the Supposed Hereditary Properties Of Diseases*. He was a man way ahead of his time, and his book showed considerable insight into many of the principles of modern-day medical genetics. On the basis of family patterns, he clearly distinguished between recessive and dominant disorders, and highlighted the association between hereditary weaknesses and environmental factors. He foresaw also the possibility of abnormal genes and even recommended the introduction of genetic registers.

Present ideas about genetics stem from the work of Gregor Mendel, a Moravian monk, who studied the subject in the 19th century, on entering the Augustian Order. After failing to become a school teacher he went, in 1853, to a monastery at Brunn where his famous experiments on garden peas were carried out in cloistered gardens. He discovered that characters existed which were transmitted unchanged from generation to generation as factors - which we now call genes - units of inheritance.

They existed in pairs and every sex cell contained one of each pair of characters. He noticed that usually only one characteristic in each pair was actually visible in the offspring. Mendel kept accurate records of his work and published his findings in 1866. No one took much notice of his results at the time, and the solution to a problem that had defied some of the world's greatest thinkers was ignored until 1900. Only then was its importance recognised and Mendel rightfully took his place as the father of genetics.

In 1902 Mendelian inheritance was shown in mice and poultry. In 1903 albinism became the first Mendelian characteristic to be discovered in humans. However, these discoveries did not explain where these genes, these carriers of inheritance, were located or, indeed, their structure. So biologists turned their attention to unravelling the next stage in the story of genetics which focused on the internal structure of the cell. Interest centred on what are known as chromosomes, thread-like bodies found in the cells nucleus. These structures had been noticed with interest when improved microscopy made it possible to see more detail inside cells.

Since these early days in the science of genetics, research and discovery have gathered momentum. In 1953 the modern genetic revolution started with Watson and Crick's nobel prize-winning discovery of the structure of DNA which answered the question about how DNA passed on genetic information from one generation to the next.

The field of genetics is exciting and relevant to an understanding of Stickler syndrome and it would be helpful at this point to give a simple basic explanation of some of the terms involved in any discussion of genetics.

Let us return to the cell, the basic building block of all living things. A thin membrane surrounds each cell, allowing substances to pass in and out of it. Most of the cell is made up of a jelly-like fluid called *cytoplasm* in which organelles - tiny structures with particular functions such as digesting food and releasing energy - are contained. The cell is controlled by a nucleus, a relatively large structure that directs the cells activities and contains the cell's chemical instructions.

These instructions are stored in substances called nucleic acids, *DNA (deoxyribonucleic acid)* and *RNA (ribonucleic acid)*. DNA, which makes up genes, holds the code which gives the instructions as to which proteins are to be made, and RNA is the carrier of information which leads to the manufacture of all proteins which form the various cells. Chromosomes are the structures into which the DNA is organised. Each chromosome consists of a single DNA molecule - which can contain millions of atoms - combined with special proteins. The DNA molecule is made up of two strands (of sugar and phosphates) which twist around each other to form a shape called a double helix - like a spiral staircase and its bannister rail - held together with chemicals called bases. There are four different bases involved: adenine (A), thymine (T), cytosine (C) and guanine (G). These bases in the DNA molecule are arranged as a code of three bases long, working like the letters of the alphabet. The 'words' used by the genetic code are called *codons,* and by varying the sequence of codons different proteins are made. As there are four bases, 64 different codons - groups of three - can be arranged.

Each codon specifies a particular amino acid or shows where a protein chain should stop or start. For example, AAG is the code for an amino acid called lysine.

There are twenty amino acids, which can combine in a huge number of different possibilities to produce all the different proteins that make up all living things. Using this simple four-letter chemical code, DNA spells out our body's life code in a message some three billion letters long. In you can imagine having an unlimited number of beads of four different colours which you can arrange in any number in groups of three, you can see how many different code messages you can make.

The second nucleic acid, RNA, is the key to understanding how the DNA is transmitted into the proteins that make us. A complex single stranded chemical, it directs protein manufacture from blueprints laid down by the body's DNA.

As we have seen, almost every cell in our body has a double set of chromosomes. One set passed on by our father and one from our mother. Cells with two sets of chromosomes are called *diploid*. Our sex cells - sperm and ovum - have only one set and are known as *haploid*. Sex cells fuse at fertilization and a single diploid cell, a zygote, is created with a full set of chromosomes.

Every species of living thing has a precise number of chromosomes in its cells. A human has 46 chromosomes arranged in 23 pairs, a dog has 78 in 39 pairs while a fruit fly has just eight chromosomes and a pea plant 14, again arranged in pairs. Each chromosome is made up of or 'carries' a large number of specific genes.

If cells are our basic building blocks then genes are our basic unit of heredity. Each gene carries certain specific genetic information - a set of coded instructions - as we have seen, relating to the composition of a protein (often an enzyme, a chemical which speeds up chemical reactions), which in turn controls the production of a characteristic, or part of it. Some characteristics are controlled by just one gene such as tongue rolling, while others are controlled by several genes working together, e.g hair colour, in humans. Human DNA stores about 100,000 genes.

As we have seen, genes exist in corresponding pairs. These are called *alleles* and are alternative versions of the same gene and are always in the same position or locus on homologous (the same) chromosomes. A dominant allele is one that is visible in the living body, be it animal or plant. A recessive allele is masked by a dominant one but is part of the genetic make-up and so will be passed on to the next generation. It will only be 'expressed' or put into action, as it were, if it is later partnered by an identical recessive allele.

Each organism's genes, therefore, contain the instructions for building its offspring, but biological reproduction is complex and prone to accidents. When the sex cells, which are all genetically different from each other, divide, a special cell division called *meiosis* occurs. This consists of two divisions one after the other. During this time the genes or alleles are mixed up or 'shuffled'. At the same time the alleles can be altered. This occurs accidentally and is called *mutation*. If a mutation occurs in a sex cell it can be passed on from one generation to the next. Mutations are a source of variation in living things and have allowed evolution to take place, but mutations are not always necessarily for the better or worse, most have no effect as they do not involve genes.

Each of us has in our cells genes that have gone wrong, i.e. mutated. About 100,000 genes determine our physical characteristics and attributes, but everyone has at least five or six that have become altered in a dangerous way. These are genes for genetic diseases. On average about 10% of the population has or will develop an inherited ailment of some kind.

There are three main forms of genetic disorders: dominant, recessive and X-linked. The latter occurs because the defective gene is located on a sex-determining chromosome. Of our 46 chromosomes, two, known as X and Y, determine what our sex will be. Females have two X chromosomes, males an X and a Y. In the sex-linked disease it is usually a defective X chromosome that is passed from a symptomless mother to her son who will be a sufferer of the defect. Any daughter she may have could be a carrier but would also be symptomless. Examples of common X-linked diseases are haemophilia and muscular dystrophy - the most commonest being colour blindness which affects 8-10% of all males.

A recessive disease can only show in a child or adult if two 'carriers', who may not have the disease themselves, produce offspring. There is then the chance that any child they have will receive the defective gene from both parents. In that case a child is born with the disease as there is no 'dominant' normal gene to mask the recessive defective one. We all carry several such genes but luckily only a small fraction of carriers with the same defective gene meet and marry. Common recessive genetic disorders include cystic fibrosis and PKU (phenylketonuria).

Now we come to the dominant disorders of which Stickler syndrome is one. These disorders do not rely on two carriers meeting but are simply passed on by the carrier to their offspring at a chance of 50% This is because as an affected parent can give only one of two genes to their offspring, one defective or one normal, each of their children has a one in two chance of being given the defective gene which will then show up as it is dominant over the normal gene.

Early research carried out in America in 1979 suggested Stickler syndrome may be due to a collagen defect. It has since been shown that the gene for type 11 collagen called COL2A1, which is found on chromosome 12, could be responsible for Stickler syndrome in some families. It did not prove COL2A1 was at fault but suggested that it or one nearby was a likely candidate for study. Although this is consistent in that most of the tissues affected by Stickler syndrome are rich in type 11 collagen, which is an important component of cartilage, nucleus pulposus in the vertebrae and vitreous humour, the data is inconclusive as I write.

So lets re-cap, when a baby is conceived and begins to grow in the womb it has a soft cartilage skeleton before the bones are developed. If the wrong collagen units are made and the proteins curl up into the wrong shape, the Stickler syndrome baby may develop faulty shaped bones. In the head this can cause a cleft palate and a flat face with a small lower jaw. The bones in the arms and legs often have big ends, leading to large loose joints. If the lens of the eye is the wrong shape this causes shortsightedness (nearsightedness) or myopia. This is because the eye is big.

One way of connecting Stickler syndrome to COL2A1 is by DNA analysis in families where there is evidence of many affected members. A group of medics, led by Ruth Liberfarb, in the Department of Medicine and Paediatrics at the John Hopkin University School of Medicine in Baltimore USA, set out to answer the question: Do mutations in type 11 Collagen cause Stickler syndrome in some or all affected families?

DNA from affected patients were compared to normal relatives and it was discovered that in most of the five 'Stickler' families studied there seemed to be an abnormal COL2A1 gene in the affected members. This suggested that, at least in some families, the mutation causing Stickler syndrome affects the COL2A1 gene. However, investigations were hampered by the difficulty in obtaining tissue from some affected individuals. In their findings published in 1988, the researchers concluded that for the time being, a mutation in COL2A1 can only be explained in some families with Stickler syndrome and not all families.

It has subsequently been shown that different families with Stickler syndrome have different errors in the DNA code within the COL2A1 gene, others may be in COL5A1 or COL11A1. Many errors seem to occur because a 'stop' codon had taken the place of a 'go-ahead' codon. This means the collagen molecule has been cut off too short and so will not fit with others to make a strong structure. In some families one code has been replace by a different one. This twists the shape at this point and so prevents a proper fit.

The first error was discovered, in 1991, by a group of medical professionals working at Philadelphia USA. An error altered a building CG code and converted the codon CGA to a 'stop' codon. It was predicted that this would decrease the strength of the amount of normal and abnormal collagen II molecules produced by the normal and defective genes.

In 1993 the same medical team reported a second change resulting in a 'stop' codon in another affected family. From these case histories there was no doubt that both families were typical of Stickler syndrome. One family had six members with myopia, retinal detachments and osteoarthritis. The other family had affected individuals with cleft palate and typical skeletal changes. As in other collagen disorders each family had a unique mutation, and it is interesting to note that although errors introducing a premature stop codon are unusual in collagen disorders in general, it may be the norm for Stickler syndrome.

In 1994 Martin Snead and associates studied a series of Stickler syndrome patients to try and distinguish between vitreo-retinal phenotypes and linkage to COL2A1. As type 11 collagen is the major component of secondary vitreous and incapable of re-formation, COL2A1 mutations might be expected to produce congenital and permanent abnormalities of the vitreous structure. In this study the patients underwent a full clinical and ophthalmological examination by Martin Snead. Patients were identified from the database of patients referred to Addenbrookes Hospital in Cambridge, UK, and classified into two groups - those with the congenital vitreous anomaly (type one) and those without (type two) and both groups were subsequently tested for linkage to the COL2A1 gene. A total of 97 affected patients were examined - 69 from 20 unrelated Stickler type one families and 28 patients from 4 unrelated Stickler type two families.

The type one families showed a linkage to COL2A1 and findings were consistent with the clinical findings, a small non functioning vitreous gel occupying the retrolental space or no gel structure at all. This feature is evident from birth in these patients and remains unchanged throughout life.

In contrast, none of the type two patients showed the vitreous retrolental abnormality. However the vitreous gel structure in type two patients was also congenitally abnormal with very limited and random fibrils, tracking through the entire vitreous cavity.

These results provide evidence to support at least two distinct genetic subgroups in Stickler syndrome. As Martin Snead and associates were able to clearly link families with congenital vitreous abnormalities to the COL2A1 gene, it was proposed to clinically classify this group as type 1. Those Stickler syndrome with congenitally defected vitreous gel structure, but *without* the type 1 anomaly have been classed as type 2. This classification will help in the search for the type 2 gene or genes and linkage of these families to other candidate genes in being examined.

Of course this is only the beginning of a new and exciting era in genetics. Mankind understands only a fraction of the code for life, and 'reading' genes has become possible on a large scale only recently. The rough guide to the genes, called a map, is discovered by tracking the way in which genes are inherited. These maps will provide the key to identifying genes responsible for disorders such as Stickler syndrome, the starting point for finding their cause, and a possible cure. So far about 2,000 genes out of the 100,000 genes have been identified and mapped. More research needs to take place before the whole mystery is unravelled. It is only then that its connections with diseases can be fully understood.

One very important benefit of knowing about, and understanding Stickler syndrome is that patients and their families can be alert for the first signs of a problem, such as a retinal detachment, which can be successfully treated if caught quickly. More importantly, if it can be identified who is at risk, preventive treatment can be given.

YOUR QUESTIONS ON GENETICS ANSWERED

What makes up our characteristics?

Our characteristics are due to certain chemicals in the body which are called proteins. There are thousands of these chemicals and each has a unique shape which allows it to do its job properly. I think of proteins basically falling into two large groups.

1. Tiny ball shaped ones which carry out chemical jobs in the body and are called enzymes. They promote reactions like making energy from the food we eat or carrying oxygen in the blood.
2. Long thread-like or stringy shaped ones which make up the structure of the body.

How do errors occur?

The DNA in a gene acts as a pattern to direct the making of its unique proteins out of simple chemical units. These units are called amino acids. There are only about 20 different amino acids which make up the thousands in each protein, and it is the order in which they are joined in a long molecule that is important. Each one has its own shape and character, which in turn causes the protein to curl up into its special globular shape, or twist around into a fibrous rope.

DNA can undergo a change. This change is called a mutation.

It will alter the message and this then causes the wrong amino acid to be put into the protein. As all these proteins work by having a certain structure, the wrong shape can cause a defect in our body.

Errors or mutations are occurring naturally all the time in all living species. Some cause good effects as well as bad effects, and they are essential in the long term to any species and plant or animals so that it can change and adapt to live in new environments. Errors happen at random. There was *nothing* you or your ancestors could have done to avoid having them.

If a protein is the wrong shape it will affect the way the body works. For example, if one protein needed to clot the blood does not function, the person will have haemophilia. If a fibrous protein is the wrong shape it means that the structure of some parts of the body are weak. This is what happens in Stickler syndrome when one of the collagen proteins has been altered.

What is meant by a dominant trait?

A dominant trait is one which has obvious results when a person possesses two alternative forms of a gene. Therefore a person with an autosomal dominant trait possesses the abnormal, or mutant gene which causes the disorder, as well as the normal gene. There are over 2,000 separate conditions and traits that can be classified as autosomal dominant, and in dominantly inherited disorders - like Stickler syndrome - a person only needs one altered or abnormal gene to show the defect, and will hand it on to approximately half their children. A condition such as Stickler syndrome, which is inherited by an autosomal dominant trait, affects both males and females.

What are the genetic implications?

I am amazed at the number of letters and telephone calls I receive from those affected by Stickler syndrome who are still unaware that this is a genetic condition. I do not blame the medical profession, but research has shown that some Gps and consultants are similarly uninformed.

Sometimes the patients or their families do not understand fully that, as an inherited genetic condition, it has been passed to them from a parent and that they in turn can pass it to their children. All too often it is easy for them to understand that they have inherited the condition from a parent, but they are shocked when it is pointed out that they too can pass it on to their children. This all goes to prove that lack of awareness is a major problem.

The patient must be made aware that Stickler syndrome is a genetic condition. Only then can its implications be carefully explained to the patient and any worries discussed with the whole family. From my own research I have found that where one member of the family has been diagnosed, further investigations have proved that three or four living relatives have been diagnosed too. A subsequent delve into the family history has revealed that many deceased members may possibly have been victims, and suddenly unexplained difficulties within that family unit have become clear.

Aunt Maud's arthritic knees, and Uncle Bill's blindness take on a whole new dimension. In some families as many as 12 members have been identified following one diagnosis. I even came across one family where 15 affected members were identified after consultation with a geneticist, and we can all imagine the emotional effect that would present to a family. Yet one consultant even went as far as to tell one member of the Support Group that he considered the condition so rare that there were only about six cases in the UK. In contrast Addenbrookes NHS Trust Hospital in Cambridge have 179 affected persons currently on their data base.

Is Stickler Syndrome always obvious in an affected person?

In some cases the individual may appear perfectly healthy and have no obvious physical signs even though the patient is known to carry the disorder because he or she has an affected parent and has produced an affected child. No evidence of the condition may be found even after the most thorough clinical examination. In other cases it is very obvious. A geneticist will construct a family tree beginning with the first person in the family to be diagnosed with Stickler syndrome. This person, referred to as the proband, will be carefully questioned about the health of all maternal and paternal relatives commencing with brothers and sisters. All relevant information will be entered on the family chart and other members examined, to discover if they are suffering from the condition. Often a number of unexplained non-specific complaints take on a whole new dimension.

Can Stickler Syndrome affect a person who hasn't got an affected parent?

As I have already said, in autosomal dominant traits each affected person usually has an affected parent. However, there are a few exceptions where the disorder may suddenly appear in one generation without a previous history. Genetic conditions do have to start somewhere, and this can be alarming for the family. Occasionally this has been explained by a delicate matter of illegitimacy, or adoption, or that one parent is so mildly affected that it has not been detected.

Mary, an American woman, is quite badly affected by the condition, as are her three children. Discussions with her parents revealed nothing of significance and proved them to be perfectly healthy. Suddenly her mother broke down and revealed that Mary was adopted as a child because her natural mother was unable to care for her and her brothers and sisters because of ill health. An indication of Stickler syndrome perhaps? Unfortunately Mary has been unable to trace her family, but the search goes on.

In most cases, the likely explanation, however, is that a new mutation has occurred and this is not considered to be so rare as previously thought. This is equivalent to a 'sport' in horticulture - the sudden and unexpected appearance of a new variety. This gene can then be passed on to future generations through the new person affected by Stickler syndrome. Why this happens has not yet been discovered, although there are some interesting ideas about why mutations occur, e.g natural radiation, but I am sure in years to come researchers will know a lot more about why an error occurs.

This happened to another family. When their third daughter Michelle was born with a cleft palate, no nasal bridge and a short jaw they were shocked and alarmed. Initially Pierre-Robin sequence was diagnosed, then a geneticist identified Stickler syndrome. Extensive investigations revealed that Michelle's sisters, parents and both sets of grandparents were perfectly healthy. A mutation had taken place.

Does one gene make just one protein?

Although one gene makes one protein and may completely control a characteristic, more often it is a number of genes which make a collection of proteins. These work together to control a characteristic. For example your height is controlled by more than one gene.

If the affected person eats a high protein diet will this rectify the fault?

Although in Stickler syndrome proteins are faulty they cannot be rectified by eating a high protein diet. All proteins are broken down by the process of digestion, and reassembled to make new proteins. The problem with Stickler syndrome is that the message to make the collagen II fibre contains an error.

Should I have children?

In many of the letters I have received I am asked if they should go ahead and start a family. Having children is a very personal decision, and one that should be taken solely by the prospective parents, but only after understanding all the implications. Because of the variable expression of Stickler syndrome it is not possible to know if a faulty gene will be inherited or to predict how severely a child who inherits the gene will be affected. Many inherited conditions can be diagnosed in unborn children by one of the several techniques such as ultrasound and amniocentesis. In families where there are at least three living affected members in at least two generations, study of blood samples may permit prediction of the affected baby through linkage studies, although this has never been done in the UK as yet. This may show that Stickler syndrome is linked to the gene locus on chromosome 12. In other families, if a mutation in the gene has been seen, this can be studied in the unborn child by taking a small sample of the placenta (chorionic villus biopsy), or growing the baby's cells from a sample of amniotic fluid (amniocentesis). However what is possible with one family, may not be possible for another and the up-to-date situation should be discussed with a genetic counsellor.

There is also the other option of adoption, surrogate motherhood or artificial insemination by donor. These again should be discussed with a genetic counsellor. Patients of child-bearing age should be referred to a genetic counsellor. If this has not happened and children are planned, the service should be asked for. Careful counselling with the patient and the family will enable correct decisions to be made in the light of the full facts of the condition and its possible effects on future generations.

Four years ago a young lady suffering from Stickler syndrome asked me whether she should start a family. I replied that it was a question I could not answer and suggested she contact her local family planning counsellor or a geneticist. Having been told all the facts she and her partner decided to go ahead and have a child. Her daughter was born two years ago suffering from Stickler syndrome but the parents say they are coping because they knew the risks and problems beforehand, and were prepared for them.

It must be remembered, though, that parents not only have to deal with their own problems but also with the stress of bringing up a child with a progressive condition. The child may need special care and attention at a time when the parent isn't well, or finding it difficult to cope, or coming to terms with failing sight or painful joint surgery. This may be particularly traumatic when the parent is weak after an operation, especially if other members of the family are unwilling or unable to offer any practical help or support. All too often, relatives shy away from anything they don't understand or that looks challenging.

What are the chances of a parent passing the condition to a child?
If a parent has the faulty autosomal dominant gene there is a 50% possibility of a child being affected, the same chance as having a boy or girl. Once Stickler syndrome has been diagnosed in a person there is a 50% chance of passing on the condition with every pregnancy.

For example, if a couple's first child is affected, the chances of the second and subsequent children being born with the condition is still 50% - having one affected or healthy child does not change the risk.

How Is life affected by Stickler Syndrome?

Those who are mildly affected say that major life questions like education, choice of occupation, marriage and having children, have only been influenced a little by their condition. However, those who are more severely affected usually say that Stickler syndrome has played a major role in all such decision taking. Choosing suitable careers has been the key to the successful management of their lives. Once adulthood is reached many have had to consider studying the best pension plans to allow for early retirement on health grounds where necessary, and making the decision to live near to transport or work.

What are other parent's reactions when they learn about an affected child?

Reactions vary and it is up to the parents to ensure their child is treated like any other child.

One parent complained that her affected child is never invited out with other families, nor asked to stay the night with friends. This can be particularly hard for a child who sees no problem and considers himself or herself 'normal'. To prevent this, relatives and friends should be encouraged to treat the child as they would any other. This will not become an issue if the parent points out any difficulties, and makes certain that a timetable of medication, if required, accompanies the child. From enquiries received, I have found that, because life can be tough for Stickler children, they are far more resilient than unaffected ones, and appear to possess an extra inner quality to cope and survive. Also, I have found the problem appears to stem from the adults not the children. Children accept one other, including disabilities, more readily than adults do. One little girl told me that her sister, a Stickler sufferer, was 'quite normal, the only difference being that she just couldn't see too well or walk as far as everyone else.'

I feel so guilty at passing on the condition to my child.

Many parents add to their own anxiety because they experience immense guilt at having passed on the condition, although most at the time did not know they had a genetic condition. One such mother with three affected children, told me that when two of her children were in hospital undergoing painful surgery she went through every operation with them, almost feeling the pain herself. She had not been diagnosed as having Stickler syndrome herself until two years after her third child was born. Sadly, she discovered she was also an adopted child so had no way of knowing about the condition nor how many of her family were affected.

For parents like this, who were unaware of the syndrome at the time they had children, there is no reason to feel guilty. It is **NOT** your fault. This seems such an obvious statement, but our emotions are not always logical. As I have said earlier in this book, the best way to overcome problems is to discuss them with your GP, consultant or counsellor as soon as possible.

However, there are some families who do know they have the condition and feel no guilt either. The decision to have a child is entirely the couples, and who is to say if it is right or wrong for them to go ahead and have a child.

Not so long ago birth defects were considered a sign of 'bad blood', or a punishment for misdeeds in the lives of past generations. Children with defects were kept secret and locked away in an institution. Thankfully, we are more advanced in our thinking today, but remnants of these mistaken feelings still remain. I have received many letters from sufferers saying, 'They are a good family, and cannot understand why this has happened to them'. I cannot stress too strongly that there is nothing to be ashamed of. Stickler syndrome is simply a genetic accident, rather like a complicated jig-saw with all the pieces there, but one or two not fitting correctly. Once a defect has occurred it is beyond anyone's control and, although it cannot be corrected, a few adjustments to your life style and an acceptance of the situation can help you to cope. It is only by talking freely about such difficulties that we can share our experiences and learn from one another.

CHAPTER FOUR

THE EYES

Before we can understand what happens to the eyes of patients with Stickler syndrome, we must know a little about the component parts of the eye and how they work.

Think of the eye as a camera. There is a lens to focus on the picture, a coloured iris which adjusts the amount of light entering the eye, and a retina which is like the photographic film. The retina, like a film in your camera, is essential. Without it we have no image to the brain.

The white part of the eye, the sclera, is covered by a thin transparent layer, called the conjunctiva. The pupil is the round black hole through which light reaches the retina. Behind the iris is the lens which is constantly changing shape to alter the focus so that distant objects and nearby objects can be seen clearly. The vitreous, a transparent jelly-like substance which fills the eye cavity behind the lens, consists of a framework of collagen fibres and hyaluronic acid that acts as a binding and protective agent for the substance in connective tissue.

When we talk of degeneration of the vitreous in Stickler syndrome, we mean that the fibres come to lie together and are seen by the patient as 'floaters'. This is often the first thing that alerts the patient that 'something is wrong'. If the retina is activated by the traction of the vitreous, then the patient may experience flashes of lights or sparks. These symptoms frequently occur in the very early stages of retinal detachment when a tear is developing in the retina. It is *essential* to be alert for any changes in the eye, and to report them immediately.

The retina lines the inside of the back of the eye, and is made up of shaped cells called rods and cones. The cones are responsible for direct vision like reading and for receiving bright lights and colours. The rods are for side or peripheral vision and react particularly to low levels of light, but they do not distinguish colours. Each has its part to play; in daylight the cones function whilst in darkness the rods are more active.

The focused image seen by the retina is transmitted to the brain along the optic nerve which acts like a television cable.

When a retina becomes detached, the light-sensitive rods and cones become separated from the tissue. The fluid that is normally present inside the eye leaks behind the tear and separates the retina from the layer behind. One consultant described the retina to me as being like thin two ply paper tissue that rubs together causing a weakness or tear. Another referred to the 'Stickler' retina as a piece

THE EYE

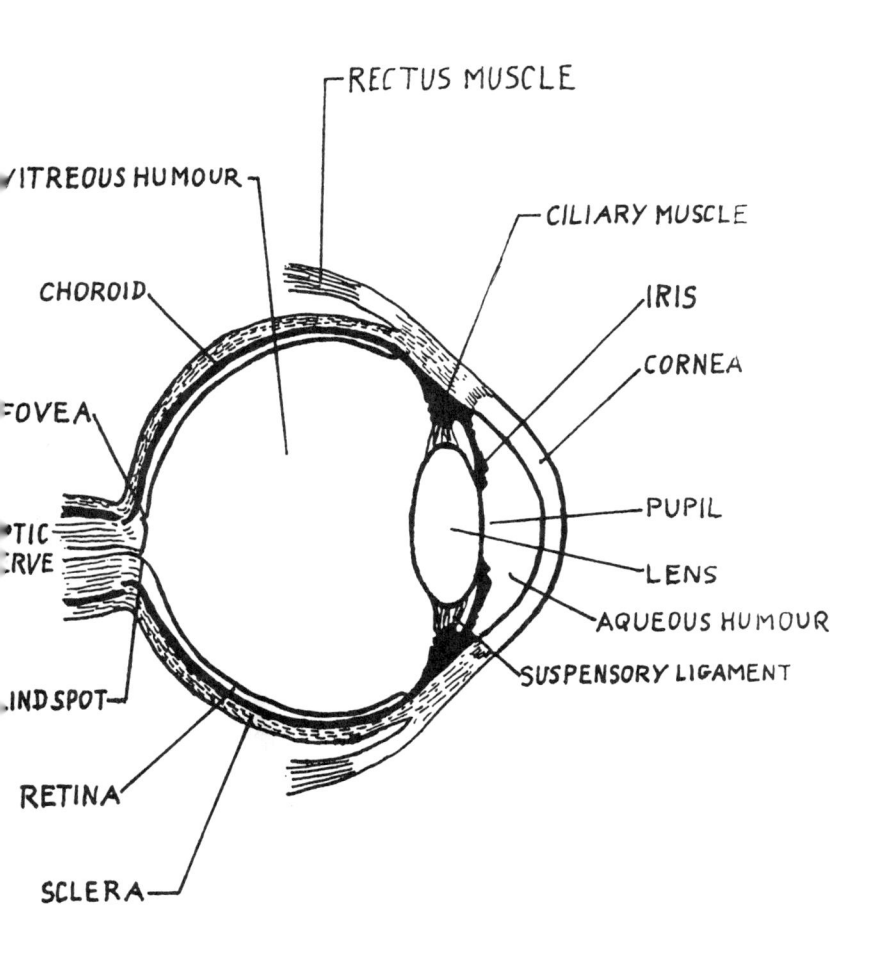

of priceless moth-eaten material that has to be carefully preserved at all costs.

Diagnosing a detachment is not an easy task for a doctor, but when he looks into the eye with an ophthalmoscope he may clearly see an obvious tear or even a fold in the retina where the patient has described seeing 'curtains'. A number of less obvious changes occur long before this dramatic stage is reached. Drops, inserted into the eye to dilate the pupil, make it possible for these changes to be seen by the ophthalmologist. However, diagnosing Stickler syndrome is relatively easy for an ophthalmic surgeon, because the changes that affect the retina are almost unique in their appearance and more often than not are the principal factors in establishing a diagnosis. These changes, unique to Stickler syndrome, include degenerative thinning of the retina, particularly along the blood vessels, and positioned far back in the retina with characteristic pigmentation along these blood vessels, called pigmented paravascular lattice degeneration. *They are not seen in any other retinal condition, or in association with myopia, and should lead an ophthalmic surgeon to the correct diagnosis.*

Thanks to modern developments laser therapy can, in some cases, prevent a potential detachment from occurring. There are two ways of dealing with this problem. The first is to heat-seal the retinal hole - like spot welding - by directing a laser beam of light through the pupil of the eye to the affected area. The scar produced seals the hole.

Your surgeon may decide to use another method called cryotherapy. This is a freezing treatment which is applied by a pen shaped probe to the outside of the eye. This freezes through to the retina hole and, as with laser, encourages scar tissue to act as a seal. These procedures are usually performed under a local anaesthetic in an outpatient clinic, and are only effective for retinal holes or weak areas.

Retinal detachments associated with Stickler syndrome can be extensive, with the separation of the two layers involving a wide area. These are extremely difficult to deal with, and *are* sight threatening. Unless expert medical attention is provided immediately this dangerous situation may lead to blindness. Stickler syndrome is the most common cause of detachments in younger people, and again should lead an ophthalmologist to suspect Stickler syndrome within that family. These detachments are generally responsive to surgery, provided they are discovered early and the correct action taken. I hope I am not painting too gloomy an outlook, but I feel it is important for those affected by this disorder to be fully aware of the problems and the importance of seeking medical attention *immediately* things appear to be going wrong.

When a retina becomes detached the surgeon must, under general anaesthesia, seal the retina to the underlying layer to prevent blindness, like sticking a piece of wallpaper back in place, to prevent blindness. An incision though the white of the eye is made to remove the fluid from behind the detachment, so allowing the retina to settle back into position. The retina is then fixed in place using the freezing technique mentioned above to seal the area. A plastic implant called a scleral buckle, or an encircling band, made from silicone rubber or sponge, pushes the outer wall of the eye. This brings it close to the retina and is not usually visible to the naked eye, as it is stitched to the eyeball's outside surface over the detached area. These bands are left in place and usually cause no problems. Any weak areas found during the operation are treated at the same time as a preventive measure.

Giant tears in the retina are common too, with large horseshoe shaped holes leading to sector detachments. Since these tears are difficult to close and present long-term complications, your surgeon may decide to perform another type of operation. This is called a *vitrectomy* and is performed under general anaesthetic. The vitreous humour is removed from the back of the eye by means of a cutter, whilst at the same time the cavity is filled with an injection of a clear substance - air, gas, or silicone oil. Tiny stitches are used to close the wound and do not need to be removed. Contrary to what people may tell you, the eye is *never* removed and replaced when any surgery is carried out. As soon as possible after surgery, and for at least 3 or 4 days after surgery, the patient is often nursed in the face down position, called posturing. The head is positioned in a certain way for the bubbles of gas, air or silicone oil to press against the retina to

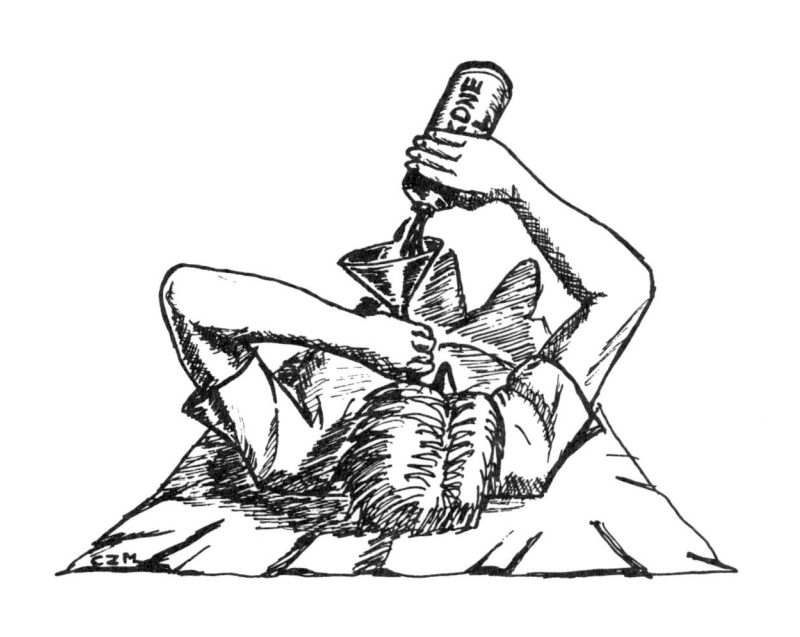

`OIL CHANGE`

close the hole in the retina. For the first few days you *must* posture as directed day and night with only 10 minute breaks each hour, except for meals, going to the toilet and washing. Once up and about the patient is told never to lie in the flat position as the substance in your eye may float to the front of your eye and away from the retina. You should *not travel by air* if you have had a gas injected bubble and it is still present. The depressurisation of the aircraft will cause the gas bubble to expand and your eye will become extremely painful. If in doubt always ask the advice of your ophthalmologist.

If gas has been used this will be gradually absorbed and disappear. The time this takes will depend upon the type of gas and the amount used. If a silicone oil is used this remains in the eye until your ophthalmic surgeon makes a decision to remove it. In my particular case this operation took place six months after it had been used. The operation was most successful as prior to the 'oil change' I had many complications with re-occurring detachments. Since then I have experienced few problems, with no new tears and the retina remaining flat.

Another symptom of Stickler syndrome is pre-senile cataracts. This is a clouding of the lens of the eye associated with increased water content. People often describe the effects of a cataract as 'looking through a mist,' or 'looking through a fine chiffon scarf.' An early cataract may have little effect on your vision and you may be unaware of its existence until your consultant mentions it to you.

Other times it will occur rapidly and the signs will be obvious. The main signs that a cataract is developing is a gradual blurring of vision, and as it progresses, the hole in the iris (pupil) looks white or yellow, instead of black.

Surgery is the only satisfactory treatment for a cataract and is usually performed at a time best suited to the patient. For example, an elderly patient may be happy to struggle along with poor vision. A machine operator may be unable to continue his work for very long, and therefore will welcome an operation sooner. It is a myth that a patient must wait until the cataract becomes 'ripe'.

However, for Stickler syndrome patients the surgeon may decide to delay a cataract operation because of other potential problems associated with the condition. The prime concern is to maintain as much useful vision as possible. The surgeon will tell you why, and you must always respect the decision.

The operation to remove a cataract can be performed under either local or general anaesthetic, depending on the type of cataract and your general health. There are several ways of dealing surgically with cataracts, and the whole procedure will take about half an hour. During the operation the lens is removed and must be replaced with an artificial lens. There are three ways of replacing the lens: with special cataract glasses, a contact lens or a plastic lens implant, called an intra-ocular lens or I.O.L for short. These I.O.L's are the most commonly used and lie either in the pupil or just behind it, to correct the focus of the eye for distance. This is not always suitable for patients with a high degree of shortsightedness (nearsightedness). The surgeon will decide and explain to the patient which is the best method. The operated eye is kept covered for 12 to 24 hours and it is advisable to wear sun glasses for a few days after the operation for comfort. Because the eye is changing shape as it heals the focus is also changing so there is no point in being tested for glasses immediately. A wait of about eight to ten weeks after the operation is the norm. This is a frustrating time but the wait is worthwhile. Unless there are other complicated problems you will need both distance and reading glasses, but if this is not the case, your surgeon will explain why.

Following a lens implant operation the vision is usually good. If you are fitted with a lens implant, the lens is a small, clear plastic lens and is never removed. The magnification is very small, only about 1% compared with the normal eye, so that there is very little change in the objects seen through the lens and the brain adapts easily to the change,

Glaucoma is another symptom of Stickler syndrome, and develops when pressure in the eye rises because fluid cannot escape. This is quite different from blood pressure and the two should never be confused.

The normal eye pressure is about 15 mm Hg, but in the case of glaucoma it may increase to twice that level. My own pressure climbed to an alarming 54 mm Hg on one occasion. When the pressure rises it is more difficult for the blood to be pumped into the eye to supply vital nourishment to the optic nerve and the retina. The condition should be treated as soon as possible because glaucoma can cause vital nerve tissue to die, and once dead it cannot regenerate.

Secondary glaucoma - meaning it develops in response to other changes - is not uncommon in Stickler patients and is characterised by a very slow change of vision. The condition is usually painless, affects the side or peripheral vision and generally goes unnoticed until quite advanced. Fortunately, testing for glaucoma is a routine part of your hospital visit. This means that it is diagnosed quickly before the loss of vision is too severe. Again, if left untreated it *can* lead to blindness.

The test is simple and painless. A gentle puff or air is blown against the eye, or a small instrument is placed gently against the eye *after* the eye has been numbed by drops. At the same time the ophthalmic consultant will look into the eye to see if the optic nerve is damaged and will also test for 'gaps' in your field of vision.

Treatment is usually by eye drops, tablets or both, and it is extremely important to use these as instructed. The aim of the medication is to lower the eye pressure to an acceptable level, but this will only happen as long as you are using the drops or taking the tablets. Successful management will not improve the level of your vision but it will prevent it from becoming worse.

Sometimes the treatment has unpleasant side effects which may be severe enough for a patient to have to stop it. The eye drops can cause blurring of vision whilst others can affect your breathing or your pulse rate. The tablets may give you pins and needles in your fingers and toes and cause indigestion. *On no account* should a patient stop treatment. If these symptoms occur, seek the advice of your doctor immediately.

In complex situations, particularly after silicone oil injection, and despite strict adherence to drug treatment, the pressure will sometimes fluctuate or remain high. In such cases a surgeon may decide to try and reduce the pressure by special laser therapy. If this happens then your surgeon will explain the procedure to you. After this procedure it may be possible for you to stop using your drops, but your surgeon will discuss the situation with you.

YOUR QUESTIONS ON EYE PROBLEMS ANSWERED

How will I know if a retina is beginning to detach?

The main signs that people experience when a retina begins to detach are flashing lights, floaters, black dots, cobwebs, or a sensation that a curtain or 'something black' is falling or moving across the eye. The most severe detachments can suddenly reduce the vision in the affected eye to almost nothing and can be very frightening for the person concerned. Early surgery is *vital*. A detachment that is left untreated *will* progress to complete blindness in a relatively short time. Because of the risk of retinal detachments, the eyes should be protected from direct injury during work or sport.

After a retinal detachment, will I be able to see?

If the operation has been successful you will be able to see, but the quality of your vision may never be as good as previously. If gas or silicone oil injection has been used, the retina will not regain full function immediately after the operation, and recovery of sight can be a gradual process, often taking up to six months.

If you are a driver, you must also remember that the law requires you to inform DVLA at Swansea, and your insurance company of any change in health or sight likely to affect the safety of your driving. The law requires you to read a number plate at 20.3 metres in good daylight, with spectacles if worn. You must also have a good field of vision. You should *never* restart driving until you have had confirmation from your ophthalmic surgeon that your vision meets these standards. Failure to do so can put yourself and other motorists at risk. Under such circumstances, you could also be faced with a situation where the insurance company declares your policy null and void with disastrous consequences financially and emotionally.

Is eye surgery very painful?

Although vital to save vision, eye surgery is rarely painful. Any pain that you do experience is quickly dealt with by the nursing staff. Eye surgery has advanced considerably over the last thirty years, and surgery for a detached retina is no exception. Approximately 80% of detachment operations are successful but in Stickler syndrome recurrences are fairly frequent, mainly because the retina is very thin and in a poor condition. Re-operation is, therefore, always possible and can tide the person over for many months or even years.

What are the signs that a cataract is forming?

As a cataract develops, you will notice a slight blurring of vision which can increase in bright light and decrease when dark glasses are worn. Headlights of cars appear like stars of light and when the sun is low in the sky it will cause dazzle. Usually there is 'ghosting', like a haze around objects, and occasionally blurring of the whole vision.

I have been told that I will have to wait for a cataract operation. Is there anything I can do to make full use of the vision I have?

If you do have to wait, there are a number of things that will help you to make the most of your sight.

1. Wearing tinted lenses in your glasses will reduce the dazzle on a bright day.
2. When out of doors wear a hat with a wide brim to shield your eyes from direct sunlight.
3. Make sure that indoor lighting is correct for your needs. Try to avoid bright overhead lights that shine directly into your eyes.
4. Try to chose a chair that does not face a window which will dazzle your view. It can be most annoying to be in a room full of people and not see who is talking to you.
5. When reading or doing any close work, have the light shining over your shoulder and positioned as near to the work as is practical. I have recently discovered the advantage of using daylight simulation light bulbs, which eliminates the 'orange' glow of conventional light bulbs.
6. Immediately report any changes to your eye surgeon. Never suffer in silence; he has your well being at heart.

I have been prescribed special cataract glasses. Are they difficult to manage?

If you have been prescribed cataract glasses, you will find that the image you see is about one third larger than normal. Because of this, glasses are unsuitable if you have had a cataract removed from one eye while the other remains normal. When wearing cataract glasses it is important to look through the centre of the lens, otherwise straight lines will be distorted, and doorways may appear narrow like an hourglass. Also objects tend to jump in and out of the field of vision if they are situated at the side of the glasses. Because of this blinkered effect it is sensible for the patient to get used to wearing glasses while sitting down. Safety is most important. When going up and down stairs take special care and always use a rail where available. Don't rush and don't worry about holding people up. Never be afraid to ask for help where needed. People are only too willing to help, if asked. It will be difficult to judge distances, especially moving cars, so it is important to seek out and use pedestrian crossings wherever necessary. It is far better to make a slight detour to the nearest crossing than to risk being knocked down crossing a busy road. It may take you several months before you feel completely confident to go out alone into busy streets and traffic. Don't worry about this. On your first day out take someone with you, and build up your confidence slowly.

What is meant by fields of vision?

This is the extent to which one can see out of the sides of one's eyes when you look straight ahead.

What is meant by registered blind?

To be registered as blind does not always mean total loss of vision.

In fact, only a tiny proportion of people on the blind register are unfortunate enough not to be able to see at all, and of these, many have been blind since birth. Also it does not mean that one day you will not be able to see at all.

According to the National Assistance Act of 1948, a person who is 'so blind as to be unable to perform any work for which sight is required,' is classed as blind. A patient's sight is considered to have reached that stage if only the top letter on the test chart, called a Snellen Chart, can be seen even when it is placed just in front of the patient. This is known as 3\60 vision, which means that the patient can see at three metres distance, whereas people with normal vision would be able to see the letter at 60 metres. Sometimes, a patient will be registered blind if rather more than this can be seen. It may be possible to read the top letter whilst sitting the usual 6 metres distance away, but in these circumstances, 6\60 vision is considered as blindness because the field of vision is also limited.

What is meant by partial sight?

Generally people whose sight is considered to be substantially impaired are registered as partially sighted. This means that, although a person's sight is poor, it is not poor enough to be registered as blind. They can usually read the top letter on the chart at the usual 6 metres, and sometimes, the next three lines.

Where do I apply for registration?

Your ophthalmic surgeon will need to fill in a form, known as a BD8, certifying that your vision is sufficiently poor to warrant registration. This is sent to your local social services department who will then send someone around to discuss the situation with you.

Is the same procedure followed for children?

Usually the same procedure is followed for the registration of children, normally after a child has reached the age of four, and the vision has been corrected by glasses or contact lenses. However, children younger than four who have an inherited eye condition like Stickler syndrome, and whose sight is severely restricted, will be certified as partially sighted, unless they are obviously blind.

CHAPTER FIVE

THE JOINTS

Although Dr Stickler, in his initial studies, found signs of disease in most of the weight-bearing joints like the knee and hip joints, symptoms varied considerably from patient to patient. A series of X-rays may show that changes are taking place at a slow and mild rate.

In general, the abnormalities are characterized by abnormal development in the way the bones have been formed - a defect in the production of protein, collagen fibrils, with premature degenerative changes, particularly involving the cartilage. In addition, hyper-mobility, or increased mobility of certain joints may also occur and this can cause the joints to be painful at different times of life, and prone to dislocation. Some people may need to modify their way of life in order to protect the joints, and prevent complications such as early osteoarthritis, which can be the result of overuse of loose joints. Like all degenerative conditions, as the cartilage covering the end of the bone wears away, leaving bone rubbing on bone, the joints become stiff, painful and difficult to move.

The difference between osteoarthritis, generally associated with old age, and joint degeneration in Stickler syndrome are obvious from the beginning, namely the marked hyper-mobility of certain joints. Many of those affected by Stickler syndrome talk of being double jointed as children, or being able to bend their thumbs into a backward position.

The fact that these changes occur in childhood, and that an irregularity of some bones may occur, together with joint swelling, may lead the rheumatologist to investigate and suspect a connective tissue disorder.

If bone problems are present at birth, then **talipes equinovarus**, or club foot can occur. In this condition the foot is twisted downwards and inwards so that the patient walks on the outer edge of the front of the foot. It is fairly easy to correct by orthopaedic splinting in the early months of infancy.

There may also be enlargements at the ends of the long bones and also on the growing part of the bone that lies between the ends and the shaft. If severe, the long bones appear 'dumb bell' shaped. If these problems are found in a young child they normally improve with age, and there is often a period of several years when the bones can appear normal.

X-ray changes seen by a rheumatologist include mild spondylo-epiphyseal dysplasia, which is a combination of an abnormal development of the spine bones, or epiphyseal dysplasia, which is a widening at the ends of long bones. If these changes are severe, then

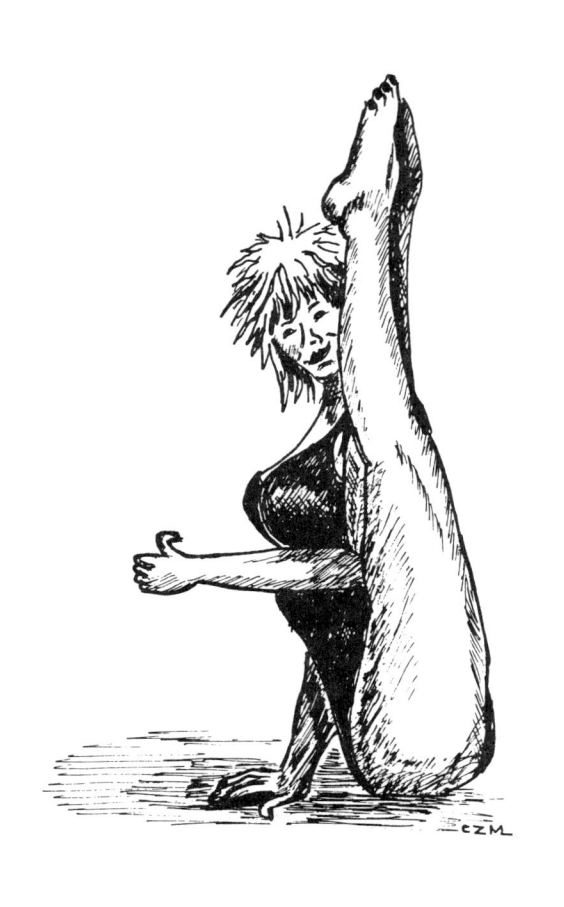

DOUBLE JOINTED!

unevenness of the spinal column or vertebrae results. The femur, or thigh bone, is usually flat and irregular and associated with a broad femoral neck. In adults, osteoarthritis of the large joints usually develops during the early 30s and 40s and tends to progress. The joints affected are usually hips, knees, ankles, and the hands and fingers. The hip is a ball and socket joint which has a wide range of movements. It is an important weight-bearing joint and is the joint in the body to be most commonly affected. It causes increased stiffness and even the slightest movement may be painful. Walking can be very difficult and even movements in bed can cause excruciating pain. When a hip is affected by osteoarthritis it gradually changes shape and the end result can be that the leg on that side becomes noticeably shorter than the other. This can make walking particularly difficult and can put additional strain on the rest of the body.

Osteoarthritis in the knees can cause a wide range of deformities. It can make the knees look knobbly and the affected person may appear bow legged or knock-kneed. Some people who are affected have difficulty in walking up and down stairs, and it is possible to hear creaking and grating noises whenever arthritic joints are moved.

The most common joint in the foot to be affected by osteoarthritis is the joint at the base of the big toe. Problems are usually caused by long term pressure generated by shoes that don't fit properly. Therefore, particular attention should be paid to comfortable flat shoes.

Considering that the ankles have to carry the weight of the whole body, it is surprising to learn that ankles are less likely to develop osteoarthritis than the hips and knees. This may happen because the ankle is only responsible for up and down movements of the foot - other movements are produced by the joints within the foot.

In the case of hands, the condition most commonly affects the joint at the base of the thumb and those at the ends of the fingers. Small, hard nodules (lumps) often form at the back of the affected joints in the hand, and although these are usually painless, they can add to the stiffness of the joints.

As most people are aware, osteoarthritis is a condition which occurs when the cartilage over the bone gradually deteriorates, becoming worn and soft and finally flaking away from the bone. In extreme cases the cartilage can disappear altogether so that bone rubs against bone, resulting in very stiff and painful joints.

Physiotherapy can help, and a painful back may respond to gentle manipulation which can provide temporary relief. A collar may help a painful neck. Ultrasound, laser or magnetic wave therapy may also reduce pain and swelling in joints.

In addition, gentle exercise may be prescribed to strengthen the area or to improve posture, but no one should ever embark on a course of exercise without discussing their plan with a GP or rheumatologist.

Many suffering from chronic pain have discovered that rubbing a sore or painful area can relieve pain. Doctors saw the benefits of stimulating the passage of non-painful sensations and produced a small pocket device that works by sending out a series of electrical pulses, which block the passage of pain messages. The technique is called *Transcutaneous Electrical Nerve Stimulation* and the device used is called a **TENS** machine. These machines have very few side effects and cost relatively little to buy, compared with a year's supply of painkillers.

Some people find the Alexander Technique helps symptoms of painful joints. The Alexander Technique or Alexander Principle was first devised nearly a century ago by the Australian actor, F. Matthais Alexander. He noticed that he kept losing his voice when working on stage and when the medical profession failed to help him he decided to investigate the problem and try and treat it himself. He discovered that he was losing his voice whenever he held his head and neck in a particular position. He assumed that the voice loss was caused by the fact that the position of his neck was squashing his vocal cords. After experimenting he found that by learning to stand properly, and by holding his head straight, his voice no longer kept disappearing.

Mr Alexander was so delighted by his findings that he retired from the stage and decided to spend the rest of his life helping others to conquer their health problems. Individuals who want to benefit from the Alexander Technique are encouraged to look at the way they stand, sit and walk. Supporters of this method are also taught to

NON RED MEAT DIET

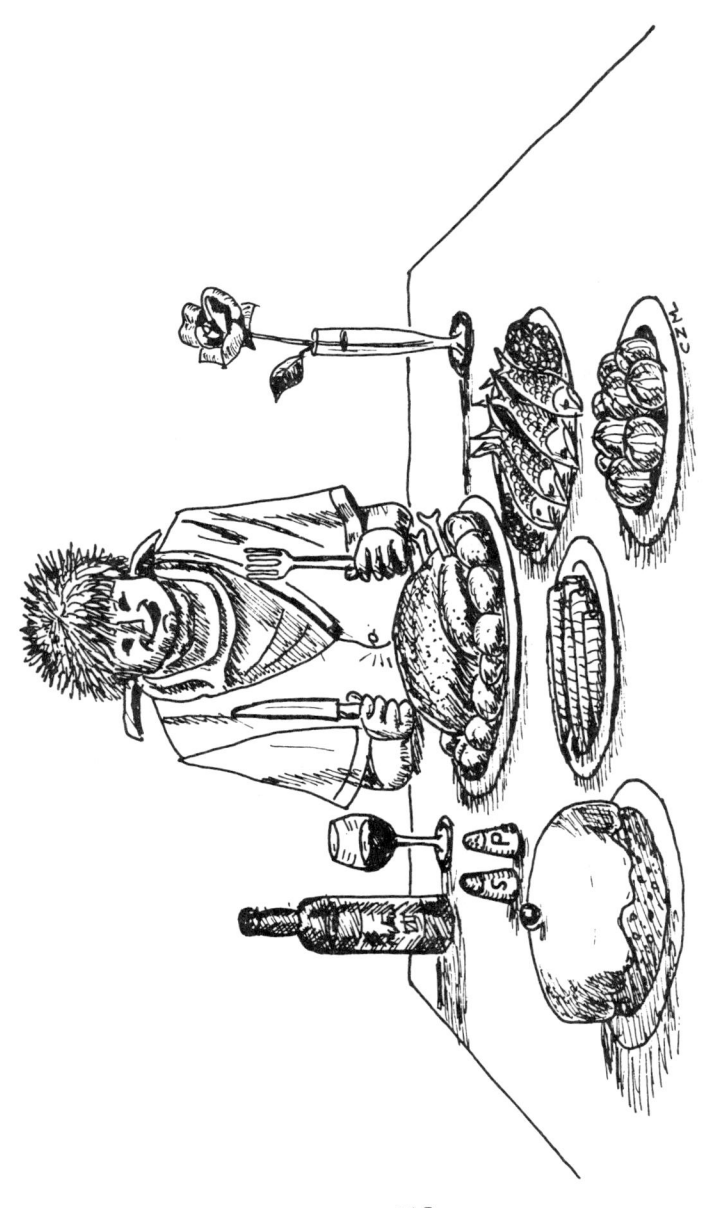

examine every aspect of their life and to pay particular attention to things like correct footwear, as these are all important factors to consider when trying to achieve a less painful life.

Degenerative joint changes can be lessened by taking the strain off the weight-bearing joints, so it makes sense for the patient to watch any undue weight-gain, and follow a sensible eating pattern. Many books have been written about diet and the arthritic, and numerous claims have been made about the importance of eating wisely. Some claim that special food supplements will help delay the onset of arthritis, others maintain that avoiding fruit will help relieve symptoms of pain and stiffness.

It appears that there are only two important dietary factors which really influence arthritis. Firstly, you are more likely to suffer if you are badly overweight, because the joints, especially the weight bearing ones, will be under constant strain. The more excess you carry the worse the problem will be. Losing weight and staying slim is essential if you are to protect the joints.

Secondly, it has been proven that you can reduce the risk of developing arthritis if you avoid red meat completely. This should help to control and minimize your symptoms. You no not need to stop eating milk and eggs, but you should limit your dairy produce consumption, especially cheese and butter.

Fibrositis-like symptoms may, on waking, be present in the lumbar area. This is an acute inflammation of the fibrous connective tissue which occurs, especially in the back muscles and their sheaths, causing considerable pain and stiffness. This can vary from very mild, lasting about 5 to 10 minutes after rising, to a severe case lasting an hour or more.

Some sufferers experience the symptoms during cold and damp weather too, but all should be prepared to experience pain the day after overuse of the joints. Others find that a spell of warm humid weather has an adverse effect on joints, and have found that doubling their in-take of fluid can help to alleviate the situation.

Your GP or rheumatologist may prescribe pain-killers to help you to manage your life. A person affected by joint pain should never buy any preparations without the advice of a medical professional, as some may make the joint situation worse. Paracetamol can relieve pain and reduce fever, but has no anti-inflammatory benefits. The maximum adult intake should not exceed 4 grams per day. If you have been prescribed anti-coagulant drugs for another disorder, then Paracetamol should not be taken.

Another group of tablets that may be prescribed are NSAID'S - *non steroidal anti-inflammatory drugs*. There are many varieties on the market and your consultant will start you off on a mild one like *ibuprofen* at first. This relieves pain and mild inflammation and is useful for treating a mild or chronic condition. As with any other pharmaceutical preparations a patient may have to try out several before finding one that is suitable to his or her needs.

Another popular anti-inflammatory drug is Aspirin, and taken in small doses (under three grams a day) can help to relieve pain. Amounts over 3 grms can create problems in the stomach and intestines such as bleeding, ulcers or nausea. Taking aspirin after eating will cut down on the amount of discomfort suffered, but if you have a known gastric disorder avoid taking aspirin. Aspirin is available without prescription, but it should be used sparingly, and with the full knowledge of your GP and its potential side-affects.

Once a preparation is found to help there is no need to take it all the time, only when joints are especially painful, such as after a shopping expedition or gardening.

Patients should be encouraged not to get into the habit of swallowing a tablet every time they feel a twinge. If taken in excess, over a period of time, some preparations can cause side effects. For example, they can cause kidney and liver damage or poison the body, causing anaemia and a blueness of the skin and lips. Also, if a patient does resort to drugs on a regular basis, the prescription may become less effective when a particularly severe 'flare-up' occurs. Some of these drugs do have nasty side-effects, so their use should be carefully monitored by your GP or rheumatologist. A patient should *always ask if there are any side-effects when a new drug is prescribed, and if so, what they are.* Doctors will be honest, if you ask. Any changes in the patients condition like nausea, vomiting, sickness, indigestion or ringing in the ears should be discussed with the GP or rheumatologist at once.

In 1950 new drugs, developed by three researchers, E.C. Kendall, R. Reichstein and P.H. Hench of the Mayo Clinic, were introduced and hailed as the wonder drugs of the century. For their work in showing that these hormones would suppress symptoms of inflammation and allergy they were awarded the Nobel Prize. These drugs are known as Corticosteroids or ACTH - Adrenocorticotrophic hormone or corticotrophin. This is a hormone produced by the pituitary gland and acts to stimulate adrenal, thyroid and sex glands to produce their own hormones. When it stimulates the adrenal glands, a group of hormones is produced called corticosteroids or steroids.

Rheumatologists rapidly seized on these drugs for their effectiveness in treating inflammation, but soon disadvantages began to emerge. It was found that steroids could, in some cases, lead to thinning of the bones, stomach troubles, high blood pressure, skin disorders and a swelling of the face and body. Yet despite all the side effects, these tablets, administered carefully with correct medical supervision, can be most advantageous, especially in selected individuals and where the problem warrants them. Anti-arthritis steroids are marketed under a variety of names, but the drug most usually given in tablet form is ***prednisolone***. Steroids do not cure; instead, they suppress the pain and inflammation of arthritis. Sometimes a patient is advised to reduce the dose, which may give rise to a paradoxical effect, called steroid fibrositis, leading the patient to believe that the original arthritic condition is returning. Do not come to this obvious conclusion but see your doctor immediately and he will assess your particular case. Doctors today are more approachable, so make a friend of your rheumatologist and discuss problems as they arise. Watch for any weight increase too. Prednisolone sharpens the appetite as well as encouraging the body to retain more fluid.

A 'one-off' localised steroid injection into an offending joint or into the soft tissue surrounding a joint can bring immerse relief for the patient in total agony from joint pain. One injection has left me almost pain-free for up to six weeks, and as pain and inflammation is relieved, mobility is increased.

If drug therapy and physiotherapy fail, you may feel that a replacement joint would be the answer. But like other forms of treatment, the advantages of an operation have to be weighed against the disadvantages. There are several factors to take into consideration, and if your surgeon has suggested surgery, then he will discuss the situation fully with you. Surgery is usually the ideal solution when treating a localised joint problem, but not the answer when several joints are involved. The joint may not be easily accessible to the surgeon, or there may be some technical reason why a joint cannot be replaced. Another consideration is the patient's age.

A SURGEON CAN REPLACE A DAMAGED JOINT

Since the 1960s surgeons have been replacing arthritic hips with artificial ones, and today hip replacement is commonplace and immensely successful - over 85% - but some patients are disappointed. Some people expect to be 'cured' overnight, but because of other medical conditions these people cannot expect to be 100% fit. If your rheumatologist suggests surgery, then it is important to establish precisely what you can expect to gain from the operation. Your doctor will be perfectly honest, but often patient-doctor communication is overlooked. It is important to establish a good patient/doctor relationship from the outset.

The operation to remove and replace an osteoarthritic hip joint - an *arthroplasty* - is relatively safe and straightforward to perform. A metal and plastic replacement hip joint is glued into the patient's bones. Most patients can stand up a day or two after the operation and are walking within two or three weeks. Advancements are constantly being made in the design of the joint replacements, and in particular in the type of materials used to provide an effective life-long replacement. Some can last through fifteen years of relatively active movement.

Another operation performed to regain pain-free mobility is *arthrodesis*. This involves pinning the joint to stop any movement. A metal pin is inserted between the two halves of the joint, followed by 'planting' chips of bone - taken from some other part of the body - into the joint space. These chips produce more bone tissue which will eventually unite the pinned joint, rendering it immobile.

Both operations result in a pain-free joint, and a patient will need to do special exercises and physiotherapy to build strength in the muscles. After any joint operation special care must be observed to ensure that the correct posture, and distribution of weight, will enable the other joints to remain healthy.

Joint replacements are of course the ultimate in orthopaedic surgery, but other operations are equally effective. Very painful wrists and foot joints can be helped by a *Resection* This is simply a removal of the offending joint. It sounds rather crude but, although it is one of the oldest surgical procedures for arthritis, it can be extremely effective.

Where the joint surface has worn away excessively, or where a deformity has occurred, another procedure, called a *Osteotomy* can prove most helpful. This means that the joint needs to be re-aligned, and a piece of bone is removed from the troublesome area and the bone re-set at a different angle. It is extremely successful in reducing pain, although not suitable for all joints. Sometimes the benefit lasts only a short time, but it may be a means of deferring the need for more major or replacement surgery.

Occasionally a rheumatologist may feel it necessary to try to increase the firmness of a joint, by stiffening it permanently. This operation is called a *fusion*, and is designed to make a joint pain-free and strong, but at the expense of flexibility. Sometimes it is more acceptable to cope with a stiff wrist or knee and be free from pain, than to be mobile in agony. Fusion can also be performed on the hips and spine, and despite its limitations, is useful in a few cases, although it is not usually the first choice when treating hips or knees.

In general, a rheumatologist prefers to avoid spinal surgery. Sciatica, for example, which is produced by a spinal disc slipping out of line and pressing on the sciatic nerve, is best treated by rest and manipulation. Interestingly, recent research has shown that the fruit of the South American papaw tree contains an enzyme called chymopapain, which can be injected into the spine where it digests away the protruding section of the disc, thus relieving pressure on the nerve. Positioning the needle requires the skill and expertise of a consultant of course, but the success rate is about 60% - the same rate as a major surgical operation to remove the offending disc. However, the long term benefits of this procedure are still being assessed, and the up to date situation should be discussed with your consultant.

Although I have outlined, for your interest, some of the available surgical techniques, no decision to have an operation to relieve painful joints should be taken lightly. Orthopaedic surgeons are not magicians. They may be able to relieve some pain or improve the look of a awkward joint, but it must always be remembered that once there is deterioration there will always be some pain or awkwardness. Again it is a case of accepting your limitations, and making the most of what you have.

YOUR QUESTIONS ON JOINTS ANSWERED

X-rays show I have the early signs of osteoarthritis. What symptoms can I expect?

The three main symptoms are pain, stiffness and swelling. Pain is the most common symptom and can vary from a dull and persistent ache to a sharp gnawing pain. This is usually worse after joints have been used, which means at the end of the day.

The pain is produced when pain endings in the bone and ligaments are stimulated. The dull, deep general ache in and around the affected joint is caused by changes in the pressure within the bone, which is the result of the joint failing to function properly. The sharper, more acute pain is usually produced when a ligament catches on or is stretched by a piece of irregular bone in the joint. Stiffness, which is usually worse in the mornings or after any period of rest or inactivity, is worse if you spend a long time in one position.

Swelling can occur when fluid accumulates, particularly in the knee joints and around the finger joints where nodules may appear.

Any advice on how best to cope with joint pain?

Pain, which can range from mild to severe and can curtail physical activity, can in the majority of patients, be relieved by rest. This can be extremely annoying, especially when the affected person is trying to lead a 'normal' life or to keep up with able-bodied friends. The secret is to find your own working limitations and, as far as possible, stay within that level, although I, for one, am only too aware of how difficult this can be.

Pain can be most uncomfortable, agonizing or downright torture, sapping every ounce of your already reduced strength and reducing even the strongest of men to tears. However, if you try to look upon pain as a necessary evil, it may help you to come to terms with continual anguish. Learn to respect your pain, and instead of looking upon it with suffering, consider it to be a friend, an essential part of your natural bodily system - a sort of early warning radar that something is going wrong, if you like.

We would all welcome a life without pain, but can you imagine how difficult life would become for us? If you placed your hand on a hot plate, you would not feel it burning through your skin. Imagine the damage that could be done by drinking a boiling hot cup of tea. Even a thorn in your finger could cause a dangerous blood infection, and you wouldn't be aware of it until it was too late. Joint pain is warning you that to pursue your activities could cause permanent damage to your joints, especially if the cartilage has deteriorated to such an extent that bone is rubbing against bone.

Most people who are in constant pain thankfully develop a high pain threshold, because they know it is going to be there. Somehow they 'condition' themselves to accept it as part of their prevailing situation and learn to cope. Finding yourself an interesting and absorbing hobby to occupy your time can help. I often 'lose' myself in a piece of writing and, whilst absorbed in my work, barely notice my constant back pain. Reading a thrilling novel can also help. If you still have enough vision, model building is an absorbing hobby, although watch your posture, and do not overdo it by sitting too long in one position.

There is one consolation. People who are in constant pain appreciate its absence, however brief, far more than a symptom-free person.

Varying your activities during the day can help to alleviate some of the pain. I try not to sit, stand or walk for too long without a change of activity. This can be difficult when you are enjoying yourself or are absorbed in what you are doing. Sometimes circumstances, like a visit to a concert or attending a lecture, can prevent you from a change of activity. Resorting to a simple unnoticeable exercise may help - like tensing and relaxing a painful muscle. There will be more information on simple exercises in Chapter Ten. When I finish writing a chapter of a book, I often wonder how on earth I am going to get up from the chair. I have overcome this problem by setting a kitchen timer for an hour and placing it at the other end of the room. On my way to switch it off I do a few simple stretching exercises, or walk up and down stairs once, before returning to my word processor.

During the day I also take a rest with my feet up and, if I fall asleep, I count that as a bonus. I find a warm bath also helps to alleviate my pain and increase my mobility. Also I make sure that I never get cold. A pair of gloves is a must in winter, so are a pair of wool-lined inner soles for my shoes. Watch out for draughts from a window, too.

It is a case of managing your own life, being in control, and being prepared to accept an 'off day'. Practise looking upon an off-day as a bonus - a day when you can rest and catch up on reading, knitting or listening to music. I usually spend these days catching up on my talking books, or thinking through ideas for my next book and putting them onto a cassette tape.

If you have a special event or function to attend, then be sensible and rest the day before, to make sure that you are in 'tip-top' condition. I know this doesn't always work, because we have no control over our condition, but at least we are giving ourselves the best possible chance. Try not to arrange events on consecutive days, and always follow a 'busy' day by a less active one.

What are the first signs of joint degeneration?

Most families I have contacted where joint degeneration is present, have told me that, like my experience, the first signs to occur in childhood were unexplained pain and stiffness. This was particularly noticeable during or after exercise or the day after using the joints.

Severe symptoms have frequently led a doctor wrongly to diagnose juvenile arthritis in the child at a young age. Complaints of aching knees or other joints should be taken seriously in such children, who should not be forced to repeat activities which cause undue stress. Sports should be carefully chosen avoiding such things as trampolining or running, and sports like swimming should be encouraged. If joint pains interfere with normal sleep or normal day activities, then paracetamol or aspirin may be used, but any therapy should always be discussed with your GP or consultant. Knee, ankle and wrist supports, provided by a physiotherapy or rheumatology department, may also help a child.

If I develop osteoarthritis, will I have it for life?

Osteoarthritis does not usually come and go, nor does it have an 'active' or 'inactive' phase, like rheumatoid arthritis. Once a joint develops osteoarthritis it remains so for life.

Can osteoarthritis be cured?

Osteoarthritis cannot be cured, but surgeons can replace a damaged joint, and much can be done to alleviate pain.

I would like to try a TENS machine to alleviate my constant pain. How do I go about obtaining one?

If you would like to try a TENS machine, talk to your GP, although you may find that he or she may be unaware of its existence. If your own doctor has never heard of these extremely effective devices ask him or her to arrange for you to see a consultant at your local hospital or ask him to refer you to your nearest specialist pain clinic.

I would like to try cutting meat out of my diet. What can I use to replace the main part of my meal?

Cutting out meat is easier than it sounds. Most of us are brought up to think of meat as the central part of a meal, so try to learn new ways of serving meals. There are plenty of alternatives - fish, chicken, pulses and a huge selection of fresh vegetables available all the year around. There are many cookery books for vegetarians, or why not see if your Adult Education Centre is running a course on vegetarian cookery? Don't replace meat with cheese or you could possibly end up making yourself feel unwell. Some cheeses contain quite a lot of fat and you could find yourself eating more fat than you were doing on a meat diet. Also, you might become bored and abandon the idea.

CHAPTER SIX

ORAL AND FACIAL ABNORMALITIES

The majority of babies born with Pierre Robin sequence have at least two anomalies - cleft palate and a short lower jaw. As most syndromes have more than two abnormalities as features of the disorder, it will not surprise readers to learn that over 80% of children presenting with the Pierre Robin sequence are later diagnosed as having a syndrome, of which Stickler syndrome is one.

In these babies the hard palate may be normal or high arched, or the baby may have a submucous cleft of the soft palate or a complete cleft. Sometimes a bifid uvula may be the only finding. It is estimated that between one third and a quarter of all reported cases of the Stickler syndrome have a clefting of the palate, but in some families, the number of family members with a palate abnormality is much greater. A cleft lip in Stickler Syndrome is rare. Once the condition is discovered a paediatrician will be assigned to the child, and his or her progress carefully monitored.

The symptom which is most common and most often overlooked is a subtle type of cleft palate known as a submucous cleft palate. In a submucous cleft palate, the lining of the soft palate (mucosa) is intact, but the underlying muscles are not joined across the midline. Therefore, they cannot work properly and so speech is abnormal. Early recognition is important, but frequently it is missed in infants, especially where there is no evidence of the parents suffering from the syndrome. Sometimes the only symptom detectable is a high arched palate which again may be easily missed.

The face of a new born 'Stickler' baby may have characteristic features including midfacial hypoplasia - where one jaw doesn't grow far enough forward or downwards. Other features include a flat nasal bridge, prominent eyes, a vertical fold of skin from the upper eyelid that covers the inner corner of the eye, a small button nose with little or no nasal bridge, and a short bottom jaw. Some parents describe their baby as 'looking all cheeks and eyes'. Any of these signs may be present and can be most distressing for the new parents, especially if they are unaware of the syndrome's existence within their family. However, many of the features, especially the short jaw, improve as the child grows so that the facial abnormalities can look less prominent by the time he or she starts school. However, if the facial abnormalities are severe, facial surgery with nasal construction may be required.

If a child is born with a cleft palate an operation is usually carried out at six months to two years. In certain types of cases the consultant may wish to perform the operation earlier or later.

Sometimes a second operation is required to improve speech, and the surgeon will assess each case individually and make a decision that is best for the child.

A wide variety of techniques have been described for the surgical repair of a cleft palate. There is however little consensus on the most effective way to carry out the repair, and throughout the world there are wide variations in the type and timing of the operation. In general, most surgeons would close an isolated cleft palate between the ages of six months and two years.

The main function of the soft palate is to help in the production of speech. Therefore the aim of the operation is to produce a functioning soft palate by the time the child is beginning to speak. During speech the soft palate has to be capable of touching the back of the pharynx to stop air escaping into the nose. If following the surgical repair the palate isn't moving correctly or cannot reach the back of the pharynx, air escapes into the nose giving rise to the characteristic 'nasal speech' which may be noticeable in some people with a cleft palate. It is therefore important that after surgery the child is monitored by a speech therapist to ensure the speech is developing satisfactorily. It may be necessary to assess the function of the soft palate by looking directly at it with a 'magic eye' passed along the floor of the mouth. This is called *nasendoscopy*. In addition, a special X-ray technique known as *videofluroscopy* may also be used to show the movement of the soft palate during speech. If following the closure of the soft palate, it later becomes apparent that the child is developing nasal speech, then an operation may be suggested to improve the contact between the back of the soft palate and the pharynx to stop the escape of air in to the nose. This is called a *pharyngoplasy* and is an operation which changes the shape of the throat to help speech. This is further explained in the question and answer section at the end of this chapter.

When determining the success of a particular method of cleft palate closure there are two considerations other than good speech development. These are hearing and normal growth of the upper jaw. Children with a cleft palate are prone to develop 'glue ear' due to the abnormal drainage of the middle ear into the pharynx. For this reason it is essential that they are seen by an ENT surgeon at an early stage to detect any hearing loss, or this may cause hearing difficulties at school. Of equal importance is the growth of the upper jaw. It is now widely accepted that the scarring caused by the surgical repair of a cleft palate may restrict the growth of the upper jaw both forwards and backwards. The width of the jaw is also restricted so that the upper teeth close inside the lower teeth with the result that they do not meet properly, As a result the face may look flat and the upper lip thin compared to the lower lip. Correction of this may require a combination of orthodontics and surgical repositioning of the jaws in the teenage years. This type of surgery is termed *Orthognathic Surgery*. In general, such operations are carried out from within the mouth to free up the jaws and move them into their correct positions. The bones are held in place by small plates and screws while healing progresses. Such operations are routine in maxillofacial units but are required only in a percentage of cleft patients.

When comparing results of different methods of cleft palate closure, the three main criteria therefore are the normal development of speech, hearing and facial growth. Such comparisons are, however, not easy, as there are so many variables in each case. Furthermore, when a new method of repair is introduced, is it many years before the success or not of the operation becomes known, as facial growth has to be monitored into the teenage years. Such studies are being undertaken, and it is hoped that the most effective method of palate repair will eventually become apparent.

With these considerations in mind, the contributor to this section prefers to close the isolated cleft palate at the age of nine months, carefully identifying the individual muscle groups in the soft palate and joining them together in the midline in their correct anatomical position. By waiting until the age of 9 months the individual muscle groups are more readily identified facilitating a more accurate repair. However, where the cleft palate is also associated with a cleft lip, both are closed together in 5-6 months. At the same time, the disruption to the lining of the hard palate is kept to a minimum to reduce the scarring and the adverse effect on facial growth. Depending on the width of the cleft, this may entail a two stage technique, where the soft palate muscles are closed at the first stage. This then leaves a residual hole at the back of the hard palate which decreases in size over the next year under the influence of the functioning soft palate. This small residual hole may then be closed by a minor surgical procedure, usually at the age of 18 months, in such a way as to minimise the effect on growth of the upper jaw. This technique for the closure of the cleft palate was originally described by Professor Jean Delaire in France and is becoming increasingly popular in the UK.

It is important that the cleft palate is treated by a multidisciplinary team in a centre used to carrying out this type of surgery. Such teams should work to well establish protocols and regularly audit their results, comparing then with other centres carrying out cleft repairs. In this way, and in combination with strong research programmes, the method and timing of the cleft repair giving the best outcome for the child should be clear.

Feeding can be a problem and sucking may be slow and difficult with feeding taking a long time. However, the feeding difficulties are usually far less serious than the mother assumes. Many hospitals have their own 'Feeding Policy' and this will be explained to a new mother. CLAPA - The Cleft Lip and Palate Association, suggests that a normal feeding method should be encouraged. As a lot of babies have sucking difficulties the association have found that the Mead Johnson very soft bottle, or the Chicco bottle which is slightly stiffer, could be used in conjunction with perhaps a Griptight Newborn teat, which is very soft. NUK have a soft orthodontic shaped teat which produces excellent results too. They also produce a range of vented teats which help with the wind problem. Some parents may find the Rosti soft bottle with its own plastic shovel a better option. There is no teat or bottle that will suit every baby, so parents may have to try more than one method. It must be remembered that a relaxed mother, a contented baby and a health visitor\midwife working together, should produce the best solution to the problem. A list of all bottles and addresses will be highlighted in *'Useful Organisations and Addresses.'*

Another difficulty, known as sensorineural deafness, affects the nerves of hearing and can be severe and progressive. An audiogram should be performed, so that any difficulties can be picked up early before the child runs the risk of becoming educationally disadvantaged by a hearing impairment. The most common reason for hearing loss in a young child is otitis media or 'glue ear'. This can be caused by several factors, but one of the most common is a cleft palate which can make the drainage tube from the ear 'kink' so that it becomes blocked. When this happens a jelly-like fluid that is naturally secreted by the ear is unable to drain away. The mucus becomes thicker and fills the middle-ear cavity which reduces hearing to a muffled roar. Grommets, T tubes or permanent tubes are usually inserted in the ears during surgery, and this can help the child's hearing levels until the drainage tube becomes clear.

If a child needs general anaesthesia then the anaesthetist should be told that the child has Stickler syndrome as intubation - passing a tube down into the lung - may be difficult due to the small lower jaw and limited neck extensibility. Obviously this applies to adults too.

These facial problems can be very upsetting for the parents, but many of the fears can be alleviated by talking to other parents who have gone through a similar situation.

When Stephanie was born she had a rather small chin and a cleft of the soft palate. Soon she had trouble breathing and could not suck from the breast or from a variety of teats. She was transferred to the Special Care Baby Unit where she was diagnosed as having Pierre Robin sequence. Stephanie remained in the Special Unit for two months because she was unable to suck and vomited at every feed. The feed was thickened to help it stay in her stomach and, because she was not gaining weight, a special calorie builder was added. She was fed via a naso-gastric tube until she was five months. At ten months, Stephanie was admitted to hospital for the palate to be repaired and grommets inserted into her ears as her hearing levels were low due to glue ear. After the operation feeding continued to be difficult. Everything had to be liquified. Semi-solids, bread and potatoes would still stick to the roof of the mouth and she would keep food in her mouth for up to half-an-hour, not wanting to swallow.

Soon Stephanie began to thrive and settle down. With the aid of a speech therapist, her speech gradually improved. A second set of grommets was inserted after six months, and when she was almost five Shah Permanent tubes were inserted into her ears to increase the hearing level. At this time it was discovered she was also short-sighted and glasses prescribed.

Today Stephanie is a normal eight year old - very sociable and happy. Her chin is catching up with the rest of her face, which has improved her features. The permanent tubes in her ears have been removed surgically and her hearing levels remain good. She is an enthusiastic Brownie, enjoys cycling and has won a gold medal at local level in gymnastics.

Her mother said that seeing her lying in the hospital incubator she could never imagine her having a normal mouth or being able to eat and speak properly. 'How wrong I was,' she said, 'If only someone had been available to tell me otherwise it would have saved a lot of stress and anguish for our family.'

Another family who suffered the trauma of feeding difficulties was the Haberman family. Emily was diagnosed as having Pierre Robin sequence. Her first few years were punctuated with hospital visits and at fifteen months her palate was repaired. Her mother, Mandy Haberman, first heard of Stickler syndrome from another parent whose child had been wrongly diagnosed as suffering from Pierre Robin sequence. She listened in amazement as the parent explained that her child had a small chin, a posterior cleft palate, long, knobbly and mobile joints. It was as though this woman was talking about Emily. Mandy immediately made an appointment with the genetics department at Great Ormond Street Hospital. The doctor took one look at Emily, who was now twelve years old, and said he was almost certain she had Stickler syndrome. This was later confirmed and, interestingly, Emily's records obtained from the hospital where she was born is endorsed on the very first page: 'Pierre Robin sequence, but query Stickler syndrome.' Someone had made the note, but this had been overlooked.

As a baby, Emily, like Stephanie, had difficulty taking food. Before having children Emily's mother had been a graphic designer, so when Emily was two she decided to put her knowledge to good use to see if she could design a feeder suitable for babies with sucking problems. 'I wanted to find a viable alternative to the naso-gastric tube and spoon feeding which I had found so traumatic', said Mrs Haberman. 'Also there had to be a solution to the problem of air swallowing, resulting in painful colic, which is so common among bottle fed babies.'

The development process was not easy, and the kitchen soon became a part-time workshop, as numerous ideas were tried out. On many occasions Mandy recalls taking one step forward, and then five steps back. Thankfully she persevered and eventually in 1984, with the help of a private company, the first prototype feeders were produced and tested on six healthy babies.

The Haberman feeder was first introduced in 1987 and has been extensively used for babies suffering from a wide range of problems. These vary from relatively minor ailments such as colic and prematurity through to complex conditions such as cleft palate, mental handicap and a wide range of syndromes including Stickler syndrome.

With conventional feeders, much of the sucking efforts of a baby affected by a cleft palate are wasted on compression of air and movement of feed within the bottle. The unique Haberman teat is separated from the bottle by a one-way valve. Once the teat is filled with milk it is held there and cannot flow back into the bottle. Therefore all the baby's sucking efforts are focused directly onto the contents of the teat, so even the weakest of sucks will gain results. The teat has an adjustable flow rate and the system allows the mother to help her baby to feed. Feeding time becomes more relaxed and pleasant for both mother and baby. Further information and details of this feeder and others are listed under '*Useful Organisations and Addresses*'.

Another baby who benefited from the expertise of Great Ormond Street was Laura Groves. When she was born in 1992, her cleft palate was quickly discovered by the staff at Frimley Park Hospital. On the fourth day Laura, in an incubator, was taken to Great Ormond Street Hospital in London for the day. She had a tube which went down her nose into her stomach, and most of her food was given via the tube. There she saw a Plastic Surgeon who decided that she would need an operation when she was about a year old. In Laura's case, he felt that it would be better if he removed the feeding tube as he felt that Laura would become lazy about sucking, but this made feeding even longer. Jill, had intended to breast feed, but after several attempts she had to abandon the idea, although for the first month or so she did managed to express her milk, but, gradually, owing to the problems and the exhaustion of travelling to and from the hospital, Jill's milk dried up. Jill found a normal teat on a bottle was impossible, so she cut large holes in the teat, and Laura was able to touch it with her tongue and release the milk. It took about an hour to feed her just 50mls!

After two weeks, Laura went home, but after 10 days she had to be readmitted because her oxygen levels were dropping, especially during sleep. This problem was solved when oxygen from a cylinder was piped into a head box in which Laura's head was placed when she was laid to sleep.

At age three months, Laura visited to the Cleft Lip and Plate Clinic (CLAPA) and Jill was advised to start giving Laura, at every feed, baby rice and milk, mixed to a runny consistency. This meant that Jill was able to spoon feed her and just top up with a small amount of milk in a bottle. Laura loved the baby rice and couldn't get enough of it, which certainly made Jill and her husband's life easier. Laura became so contented that she would sleep through feeds, so Jill had to set the alarm and wake her every four hours to

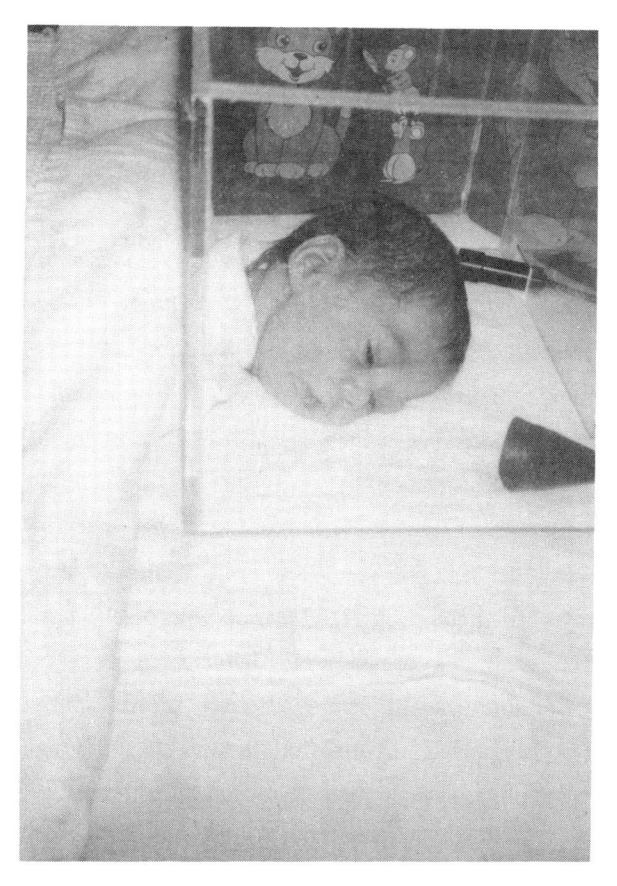

Laura Groves asleep in head box

make sure she had the required amount of milk. The Clinic also mentioned the possibility of Laura having Stickler syndrome and the family were referred to a Genetic Councillor at Great Ormond Street. There Laura was diagnosed as having Stickler syndrome, her eyes examined and glasses prescribed.

The next stage of weaning was to give Laura pureed food. This was quite easy, and she was able to have some home prepared foods, although, as with the baby rice, some of the food would come back down her nose. Because of these difficulties, it was hard for Jill to let anyone else feed Laura, which meant that she could not leave her very often.

A week after her first birthday Laura had her cleft palate repaired. For the first 24 hours after the operation she was only allowed water, then she progressed to milk and on the third day she was allowed some ice cream and yoghurt. A sloppy diet was maintained for four weeks. Her arms were kept in splints for two weeks to stop her putting anything into her mouth. Although she had never been able to keep a dummy in her mouth, she used to suck her thumb. Because she could no longer do this, she became very distressed, but when the splints were finally removed Laura had lost the need to suck her thumb.

Laura continued to make excellent progress as she graduated to more solid food, albeit soft foods. Later, when she began to talk, the services of a speech therapist were sought.

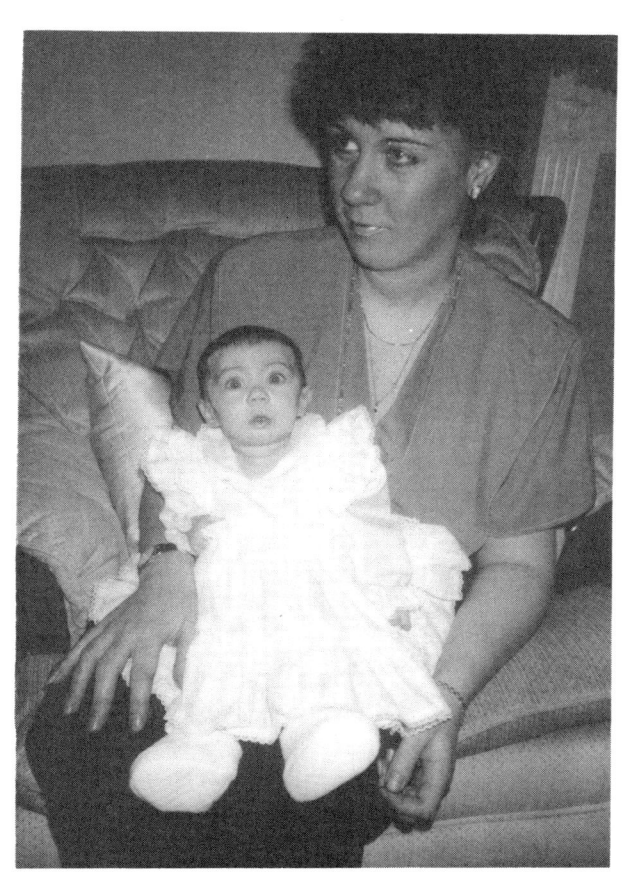

Jill and Laura

Today Laura is a happy two and a half year old and has regular hearing tests, speech therapy assessment, and eye tests are carefully monitored.

YOUR QUESTIONS ON FACIAL PROBLEMS ANSWERED

How would I know if my child had a cleft palate?

It should be picked up at the routine check after birth by the paediatrician, especially in any infant born to an affected parent, or if the baby is failing to thrive, or has a poor feeding pattern. If you suspect there is a problem, this may be checked by looking into the baby's mouth, and holding the tongue down to look at the palate. At this stage, it may be the only obvious indication that something is wrong.

Why does my baby looks so strange?

Unusual facial appearances can be very distressing for a mother, but as mentioned, features become less pronounced with age.

I had hoped to breast feed my baby. If the baby is born with a palate abnormality will this be possible?

As I have said before, each case is different and the hospital staff will advise. However, if you want to breast feed go ahead and try. In spite of sucking problems, many babies are breast feed. A nipple shield and teat may be helpful if your baby has difficulty in holding the nipple. You could also express milk and feed your baby with a bottle. Remember if you do fail to breast feed, it is not anyone's fault, some babies, without a cleft palate, have difficulties with breast feeding.

My child's palate doesn't not work well and he has been referred to a Speech and Language Therapist. What can be done for my child?

If the soft palate does not move very well this may affect talking and the speech may sound nasal. Certain sounds may be difficult to make, some may sound weak, and others may be replaced by incorrect or unusual sounds. A Speech and Language Therapist will assess how well the soft palate is working during speech, and will listen to whether a child can make sounds for which the soft palate lifts. The child will be asked to repeat words like ball, daddy and car, The therapist will also listen to the tone of voice and work out whether air is escaping into the nose, making the speech sound nasal. Some special investigations may need to be carried out to gain more information on how the soft palate and wall of the throat are moving during speech. For most children speech and language therapy is all that is required to help them learn to stop the air going into their noses at the wrong time, and to make their sounds. Some children may need an operation followed by further therapy.

It has been suggested that my child may benefit from a pharyngoplasty. What does this mean?

A pharyngoplasty is an operation which changes the shape of the throat to help speech. As I have mentioned before, when we speak, the soft palate - the back of the roof of the mouth - moves upwards and backwards, and the walls of the pharynx (throat) move forwards and inwards to shut off the cavity of the nose from the mouth. In children the palate lifts to touch the back of the pharynx. If the nose is not shut off when we speak, air leaks into the nose cavity, and speech becomes 'nasal' in tone and the air which should be used to make sounds in the mouth 'escapes' uselessly though the nose. A pharyngoplasty is designed to stop this happening. There are many different types of pharyngoplasties, and the surgeon will choose the best one for the individual problem using moving x-ray pictures of the palate and throat. He may also use an endoscope - a small telescope - passed through one nostril to view the palate directly from above as it moves during speech.

If my child has a pharyngoplasty, how long will he need to be in hospital?

The time will depend on the hospital performing the operation but as a general rule it is considered to be equivalent to having tonsils taken out. Children and adults have a sore throat afterwards and after a soft diet for a period can then go back to eating normally. Children are usually fit enough to return to school two to three weeks after the operation.

Which is the best method of feeding a baby with cleft abnormalities?

There is no best method. It is whatever suits you and your baby best. Try the simple methods first. The secret is to take your time, be patient and calm.

CHAPTER SEVEN

OTHER PROBLEMS AND WORRIES

As far as I am aware, there has been no extensive general study into Stickler syndrome. Through studying specialist articles on one aspect or another of the condition, and by corresponding and talking with families affected, I am finding that a pattern of other problems is beginning to emerge.

The major accepted symptoms have already been dealt with in some detail. In this chapter I would like to mention other known problems associated with Stickler syndrome, and outline those common to fellow sufferers with whom I have come into contact, although at this stage it must be stressed that it has not been established if these are related to Stickler syndrome. Some may be totally unconnected, but until further research can rule out their significance they deserve a mention in this book. It would be most interesting to hear from anyone who has similar difficulties, or who would like to tell me of other problems, so that a clearer picture of the syndrome can be presented, and possibly used in future studies.

Some emotional and social worries have also been outlined, and again, anyone who has anything to contribute to a future edition of the book should contact me.

MITRAL VALVE PROLAPSE.

Research has shown an increased prevalence of mitral valve prolapse in a number of connective tissue disorders. Stickler syndrome is no exception. According to a report published by Ruth Liberfarb and Allan Goldblatt in the *American Journal of Medical Genetics* in 1986, this condition was found in 45% of the Stickler syndrome patients they studied.

The mitral valve consists of two flaps attached to the walls at the opening between the left atrium and the left ventricle of the heart. Its purpose is to allow blood to pass freely from the atrium to the ventricle, but to prevent any backward flow. If the valve fails to close properly blood will flow from the left ventricle back to the atrium. If this happens, it can cause breathlessness, palpitations, (which result in a rapid and irregular heart and pulse rate), embolism and a click murmur. Although this can be frightening it is usually not serious and can be controlled by medication. However, in most cases the leak is small, symptomless and requires no treatment. Those affected can live completely normal, active lives. However, there are a few unfortunate people who do suffer serious complications. Although not within the scope of a general book like this these include mitral insufficiency, bacterial endocarditis, thromboembolism, arrhythmias and sudden death. The consultant will be able to assess the situation and advise on any necessary procedures including, in a severe case, replacement of the valve with an artificial one.

Liberfarb and Goldblatt studied 35 male and 22 female patients who had been diagnosed as suffering from the Stickler syndrome. Their ages ranged from four to 60, and 49 came from families with a history of Stickler syndrome. Twenty-five of these came from families in which two or more relatives were also included in the study.

Tests showed that of the 57 patients, 15 males and 11 females had evidence of mitral valve prolapse. In a preliminary report, published by Liberfarb and associates in 1984, the percentage of patients with Stickler syndrome having mitral valve prolapse increased to 60% when palate, eye, and musculoskeletal abnormalities were present. In the general population mitral valve prolapse has been reported to be more common in females than in males and its incidence increased with age. However Liberfarb and Goldblatt noted that in their studies with Stickler patients there was a slight predominance in females but no increases in prevalence with advancing age.

Liberfarb and Goldblatt confirmed Opitz's earlier findings that Stickler syndrome may be the most common autosomal dominant connective tissue disorder in the North American Midwest, with a relatively high frequency in other parts of the United States and in

Europe. It is also thought to be far more common than Marfan syndrome, which is found in one person in 20,000. In spite of its frequency, most physicians are unaware of the characteristic findings in the Stickler syndrome. This is a statement echoed all too often in the reports I have studied, and in the letters I have received from those having to live with the condition.

OTHER MEDICAL ISSUES

From correspondence with affected families, a small survey I conducted, and from other sources, I found that further health problems were common.

For example, many complain of gastro-intestinal disorders - non-specific gastric pain, indigestion, nausea and vomiting, gall-stones, irritable bowel syndrome and peptic ulcers. Others complain of an intolerance to certain foods, such as wheat or maize, which produce loose stools, flatulence and pain. If these symptoms exist, and persist, then advice should be sought from a gastroenterologist - a consultant specialising in diseases of the digestive tract - regarding allergy testing, a modification to one's diet, and suitable medication. Some people who have been affected say that their gastric problems have been dismissed as a 'nervous' tummy or anxiety caused through continually having to live and cope with a progressive illness. Although these are valid points, are they correct? These are all fairly common disorders which have not, as yet been connected to Stickler syndrome. Until a thorough general survey of the condition is undertaken the picture remains vague.

Another common condition identified in my research is the presence of hiatal and umbilical hernias. Again there is no information to confirm if this is connected to Stickler syndrome, but these may indicate signs of weak connective tissue.

Many sufferers have written complaining of migraine-type headaches. The most common symptoms are that they start like a tight band being pulled down the nape of the neck, or around the top of the head, accompanied by vomiting and flashing lights. Several mention a tingling around the shoulder blade area before the onset of a headache.

Others speak of suffering skin problems. In cold weather, particularly between November and February, rashes appear on the extremities about 15 minutes after coming indoors and last for about two hours before fading. Dry and cracked skin, particularly on the extremities, appears to be a very common problem. Others complain of hard cracked skin on the heels of the feet, accompanied by arthritic pain which makes walking difficult. Children often complain of cold hands and feet, which can indicate poor circulation.

A number of Stickler patients suffer from chronic urticaria - an acute or chronic allergic reaction in which red round weals develop on the skin. Others speak of allergies to food colouring and allergies to certain fibres. Many complain of boils and acne. Again these are very common complaints and whether they are yet another feature of Stickler syndrome remains to be seen. Many have undergone skin biopsies and say that dermatologists agree that something is wrong, but cannot pin-point what.

Most patients complain of becoming extremely tired, and very quickly too. Some say it is like experiencing 'hitting that famous wall' during a marathon. They are overcome by an unusual tiredness, the legs buckle and all they want to do is lie down and sleep. This is extremely annoying, and it is something that parents of Stickler children should be aware of, without being over-protective.

NOTES FOR STICKLER PATIENTS

HELPING OTHER PEOPLE TO COME TO TERMS WITH YOUR CONDITION

This is not such a silly statement as you may think. Most who are affected by this disorder experience traumas, as family and friends try to come to terms with the condition and learn to cope.

A genetic disorder affects the entire family and the hardest part is explaining a little-known condition to someone, as well as trying to get people to accept you as you are. Couples may experience a strain in their relationship when the disorder is first identified, especially if they plan to have children. Others, who first learn about the condition when their child is diagnosed may find undue pressure on the relationship, and the support of family and friends is vital to obtain a balanced overall perspective of the situation.

Grandparents may blame themselves for a child's condition, or may place the blame on the 'other family.' Some deny the reality of it, and refuse to accept that anything is wrong. All these reactions are normal.

Unaffected siblings need support too, as many may feel guilty that they haven't actually inherited the condition, or they may suffer silently believing that they might be affected and no one is listening to their worries. Put aside some time to talk to children, explain the condition and invite them to share their feelings. Ask them questions and find out what is worrying them.

For most adults who have just learned of the diagnosis nothing has changed dramatically, unless of course useful vision is lost. Nevertheless, family and friends find it extremely difficult to accept. I suppose they are scared of the unknown, and find it difficult to understand.

Most people who have experienced the condition say that other people's reactions to this newly diagnosed state fall into two groups.

The first group think it is some dreadful illness that should never be discussed and pretend the condition simply doesn't exist, and will talk about anything except your health. In some ways, this group is easy to cope with because you can gently explain you are no different now than before. Then you can proceed to 'educate' them about the condition. Show them leaflets about it and ask them to help you to reorganise your life. If they feel they are being useful they will rally round and be most supportive towards the situation.

The other group thinks life has ended for you and try to protect you, or talk about you as though you are invisible or brain dead! This can be particularly difficult, especially when a partner or someone else close to you adopts this attitude. At first family and friends may rally

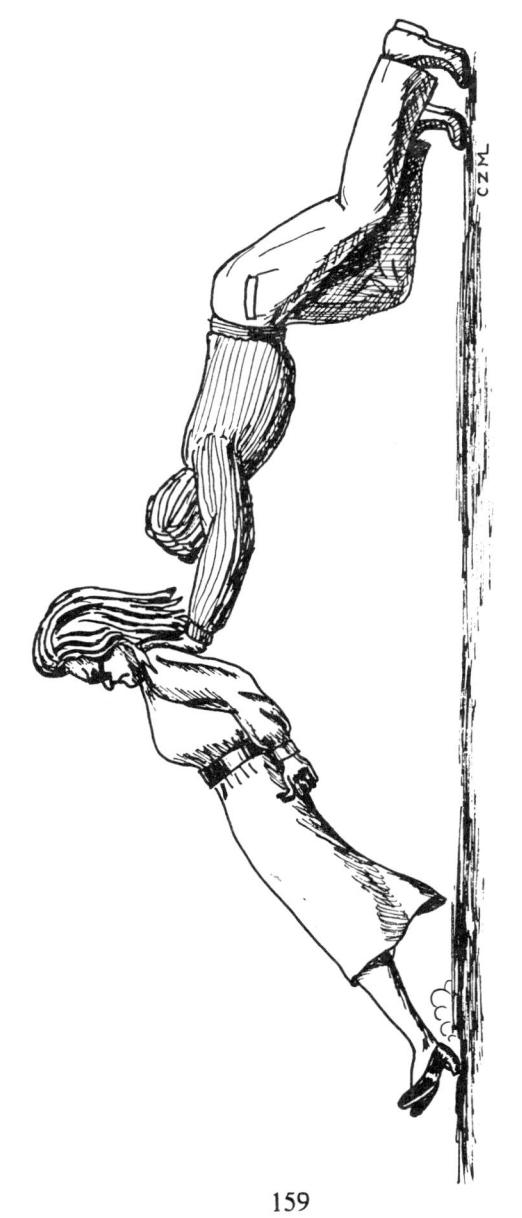

GUIDING THE VISUALLY IMPAIRED

round to do things for you, but soon they will want to lead their own lives. Then it will be harder for you to cope, but if from the outset you do as much as possible for yourself, life will be easier. Remember, it is better to have tried and failed than not to try at all. This may be a difficult period for you and everyone around you, but you should never bottle up your frustrations. To communicate your hopes and fears is essential. Speak to those close to you, your consultant or GP. If all else fails, seek the help of someone who can give you expert counselling. Only by talking through your problems can such anxieties be thrashed out and the correct action taken.

If vision has deteriorated you may need someone to guide you. Some seem to grab your arm and try to propel you through a crowd. We cannot blame them, they don't understand the needs of the visually impaired. Explain that your rehabilitation could be made easier if they would observe a few helpful hints. Then explain the following:-

1. When you are guiding me, let *me take your* arm. Never grab my arm and push me in front of you. I only need an arm as a guide, so let me walk just half a pace behind you so that I have time to adjust when you stop, reach a kerb or change direction.
2. Tell me about objects in front to me well in advance, so that I am prepared when you guide me around them. Never pull me away from an object just as we reach it, without warning.

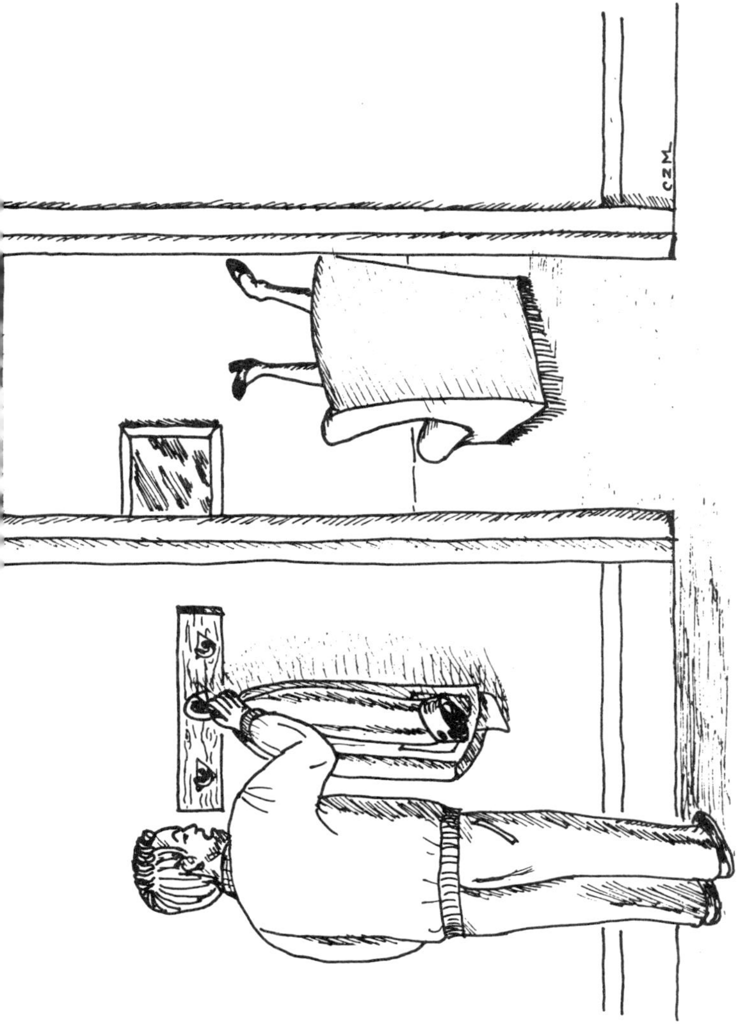

BY THE WAY, I'VE MOVED THE CHAIR!

3. When you give me directions, try not to confuse your left and right. If you are not sure, indicate by gently tapping my hand.
4. When you offer me a chair, don't just push me into it. Put my hand on the back of the chair and let me find my way around to the front of the chair.
5. Use my name when you are first speaking to me. It is so infuriating when you are in a room full of people and someone talks. Firstly, I am not certain if you are speaking to me, and secondly, I am not always sure of your voice. Don't forget most partially sighted people cannot see features clearly, so a friendly tap or shake of the hand is equivalent to a smile or an acknowledging nod.
6. If you have rearranged your home since my last visit, please tell me. Most partially-sighted people memorise familiar places and lay-outs and can become confused when things are different.
7. Please don't point to objects or pass things to me. Place them in my hand. It saves embarrassment on both sides.
8. Most important, tell me that I look smart, colourful, trendy or whatever. My self-esteem may be low if I can't see how I look in a mirror. One word of encouragement helps a lot. Conversely, if I am wearing odd socks, stockings or my accessories clash, please say so. If I spill food or have an old stain on my clothes, please tell me so that I can deal with it.

All too often problems are encountered within the family because of the extra attention afforded to a child with Stickler syndrome. Children like to help, and problems can be overcome if the healthy members are encouraged to support their brother or sister because he or she is a little bit 'special'. However, always remember that healthy children also need a life of their own, and should never be used as unpaid baby sitters or carers.

LEARNING TO COPE WITH THE CONDITION

Many families are concerned about the long-term effects of a genetic degenerative disorder. Worries can be alleviated by finding out as much as you can about the condition, and your particular symptoms. Once patients know all the facts they can accept the situation more readily, and are willing to learn to deal with it, thus giving them a sense of being in control of their lives once more. Strangely enough, I have found that a child diagnosed at birth grows up with a knowledge of the condition and is far better equipped to cope with life than someone who, in mid-life, is suddenly faced with the realisation of the condition and all its implications.

Once over the initial shock, the next step to consider is the every day management of living with a progressive disorder. Life-style should not change too dramatically at first, unless of course you are unlucky enough to lose all vision or have severe arthritic problems. Ways of coping with this are discussed in Chapter Ten. You may have to make slight adjustments in the way that you do things, but try to accept each obstacle as a challenge, a competition to find new ways of tackling some task. When you conquer that task, reward yourself, wallow in your own success. Self-esteem is very important.

Try some simple gentle stretching and curling exercises, which may be done before getting out of bed. This will certainly help morning stiffness. Protection of the retinas is most important, and all activities that are jolting and jarring should be avoided. Depending on the condition of the retina, your surgeon may recommend that you do not bend or stretch, or take part in any contact sports. It is vital that you listen to your surgeon as this will help to preserve sight.

A patient has a right to know what to expect in life, so once you feel able to talk over the situation, make an appointment with your GP or consultant to discuss any potential physical limitations or the possibility of blindness or crippling arthritis. However, I am also aware that some people may not wish to know, and your consultant will be aware of your present emotional state and may withhold information from you until he feels you are able to cope. Remember your consultant will always have your best interests at heart, although you may no realise it at first.

CARE OF A PERSON AFFECTED BY STICKLER SYNDROME

The prime concern for anyone managing and supporting a person with Stickler syndrome is to assist the patient to achieve and maintain his or her maximum level of performance, and at the same time provide a listening ear and comforting words when necessary.

One of the most common obstacles I have come across is anxiety - the constant worry of knowing that, at any moment, vision may be lost completely, or that stiffening joints are going to make life difficult, or some other problem may arise. Affected families write expressing a feeling of living with a 'time bomb' that is liable to erupt at any moment. Similarly some feel that being too complacent about the condition can lead to undue distress when something does go wrong. The answer lies somewhere between these extremes and, unfortunately, it is something that only the patient can observe.

All fears should be talked over freely with partners, family and friends, and any anxieties that cannot be resolved within your own environment should be discussed with your GP, ophthalmic surgeon or rheumatologist. But remember, they do not leave medical school with a crystal ball and cannot foretell the future. However, they can reassure the patient and, even if your worst fears are confirmed, you can learn to accept the situation and begin to build a new life for yourself. More about this in Chapter Ten.

YOUR QUESTIONS ON OTHER WORRIES ANSWERED

I find it very difficult to obtain information about this condition. Is there a way of dealing with this?

One of the major problems I have come across is the total lack of information available for those affected. This leaves the patient feeling isolated and frightened. My surgeon is wonderful and has always been willing to answer my numerous questions, although I am sure he must tire of my continual interrogation. I appreciate that not all patients have such an understanding surgeon, nor feel able to talk freely about the condition - hence my determination to write this book, and raise awareness about the condition. The Stickler Syndrome Support Group has produced a leaflet 'Stickler Syndrome - What is it?', and there are also a number of fact files on various aspects of the condition. It is up to us as affected individuals to educate as many people as possible.

When I go out with my partner, people ignore me and ask my partner how I am. How can I deal with this?

We have all heard the saying 'Does he take sugar?' And I am afraid there are many misunderstandings about any disorder, but it is often made worse by people who do not understand visual impairment or deafness. If someone asks my husband how I am and I am standing at his side, he usually replies, 'Why don't you ask her yourself? She won't bite,' or jokes that unfortunately there is nothing wrong with my tongue and I haven't lost the ability to speak. You will also find that sometimes people will shout at you or talk in single syllable language, as though they are talking to a young child. Again say politely that even if you can't see properly, or are slightly deaf, or have painful joints you are certainly not mentally sub-normal. You weren't before this condition was diagnosed, so why should you be now. It is embarrassing and upsetting to encounter this reaction, and sadly it does happen, but a positive approach to the problem can pay dividends.

CHAPTER EIGHT

YOU ARE NOT ALONE AND HOW OTHERS HAVE COPED

Most people, when they first hear about Stickler syndrome, feel a sense of isolation. Many, particular those who are diagnosed in mid-life, wonder if it is possible to lead a normal life again. The problems associated with having to attend hospital appointments and undertake many tests is worrying, especially if the patient is still in employment, or has young children to look after. Unfortunately, these worries are not made any easier by the knowledge that almost everyone the patient meets will know little or nothing about the condition. Time has to be spent explaining what the disorder is, how it affects an individual, and its implications, and this can be time consuming and distressing for all concerned.

These are the feelings and difficulties I encountered seven years ago when I was diagnosed. At one stage I wondered if there was life without operations, and when I underwent four operations in as many months I even accused my surgeon of being 'operation happy.' But very soon I realised that he was fighting a battle for *me*. Soon a pattern began to emerge and I began to fit my life around hospital appointments and 'off' days. *I started to learn to live with my condition and not for it.* This is very important. It is so easy to find yourself on a downward spiral when everything seems to be against you, and depression can easily take over. Regardless of how depressing the future may seem you *must* remain positive throughout.

Of course my eye surgeon knew about the condition and was always willing to discuss a particular difficulty, but my rheumatologist, a most respected consultant in his field, had not heard of it. Neither had my GP. Even my dentist was horrified when he realised that, despite the dental implications, he did not know about it.

At first friends thought I had misheard the diagnosis and would say, 'Oh, you mean sickle cell disease. That affects the blood, doesn't it?' Others just looked in shocked horror, then turned away muttering words of sympathy, or changed the subject completely. Sadly one or two took flight and have never been seen since. Others, mere acquaintances, have turned out to be the best friends anyone could wish for. One can certainly learn a lot about human nature when faced with a potentially traumatic situation.

Now, when I visit a new consultant, I tease and say, 'Of course, you have heard about Stickler syndrome?' and watch as some say 'no' in obvious embarrassment. Others say, 'Oh, Stickler syndrome, I will brush up on it tonight.' I know that they may know very little, or may not have heard of the condition at all, but at least I have alerted them to the condition. In fact, few have heard of it but all are intrigued and eager to learn more, which I find encouraging. I usually conclude by asking them to do me a favour and mention the condition to at least one other colleague. If we all do this, then eventually Stickler syndrome should be as familiar as the common cold.

A few years ago, I was asked to take part in a mock examination for qualified doctors who were about to take an entrance examination to become Fellows of The Royal College of Physicians. The selected 'patients' were admitted into hospital and during the day seen by thirty two doctors, who were given a rough outline of their medical history. The doctors were allowed to examine the patients and ask as many questions as they liked, but we were instructed not to reveal the name of our disorder. By the end of the day, hopefully, the doctors would come up with the correct diagnosis. This proved extremely useful in researching for this book, and at the end of the day I knew that at least thirty-two doctors would know more about this common, but little recognised condition. Amazingly, only one came anywhere near to a correct diagnosis - a young Chinese doctor - who said that although he couldn't name the condition he felt that the symptoms were consistent with that of a connective tissue disorder of some kind. He had heard of Marfan syndrome, and although my case had similarities, he did not think that was my problem. At the end they thanked me for taking part, and my rheumatologist concluded by saying that he knew it would make me happy if each doctor went away and told at least one colleague about the condition.

On another occasion, I was offered the unusual privilege of sitting in on a 'Grand Round,' case study - my own - at University College Hospital, London. These case presentations are held at most large teaching hospitals for an audience ranging from first year medical students through to consultants and professors. Usually the patient's name is not revealed, but in my case they took the unusual step of introducing me and even allowing me to sit in and answer questions after the presentation. The consultants managing my case were present and each in turn gave his story of the case aided by X-rays, test results and anything that would help doctors reach a decision concerning a diagnosis. I found this most enlightening, and even managed to see a few slides of degenerating retinas. Perhaps in future more cases of Stickler syndrome can be highlighted in this way, enabling the disorder to obtain the recognition that it so rightly deserves.

Some doctors believe Abraham Lincoln and his son Tad both suffered from Stickler syndrome. Tad certainly had a cleft palate, was tall and slender and photographs suggest he had a 'flat' face. His father was probably not myopic, since he did not wear glasses until after the age of 48, and only then for hyperopia - a U.S term for long sight. He did suffer, however, from a 'marfanoid' habitus - long slender extremities. Some professionals are of the opinion that he was suffering from Marfan syndrome, but Dr John Opitz believes that the Lincoln family suffered from Stickler syndrome. Even as I write, the debate goes on in the medical profession both in the United Kingdom and America. We may never know whether the Lincolns were affected by Stickler or Marfan syndrome, but we do know that both are connective tissue disorders. Despite all his problems, Abraham Lincoln became President of the United States of America proving that, whatever your problem, with effort and determination anything can be achieved.

I remember, a few years ago, meeting Tim, a thirteen year old from The Netherlands, who unknowingly has inspired me to continue with this book, even when I considered giving up during a period of illness and when I was unable to find the information I needed. Despite many problems he is a very 'normal', cheerful and mischievous young man. Through his mother he proudly told me that he was 'special', he had met Dr Stickler, the 'designer' of his condition, and that when he grows up, he might even become President of the United States of America, like Abraham Lincoln!

We can't change the way we are, but we can change the way we approach it, and I think we owe that much to future generations. It isn't what we have in life that is important, it is the way we use it. Never be afraid to try anything. Look on each challenge as a gamble - some you lose, some you win. To have Tim's positive approach is the best way to cope with Stickler syndrome.

Over the past seven years I have corresponded with many Stickler syndrome families, and found that most are coping, and live a full and rewarding life. Some, however, have experienced many frustrations and problems, especially before they were diagnosed. Others are still coming to terms with the trauma of it. Here I relate, with their permission, some of their stories and advice in the hope that their stories will inspire and help other families to cope in the future. Some names and places have been changed to respect their privacy.

TIM:

Tim, whom I mentioned earlier, was born in 1982 and lives with his parents and healthy older brother and sister on the outskirts of Amsterdam. It took the medical staff in the hospital where he was born a week to find out that he had a cleft palate, even though feeding was difficult and his mother told them his throat 'looked strange.' After much persuasion and pleading she managed to get the extra attention he desperately needed. By this time Tim was a very sick baby with double pneumonia and pleurisy caused by milk entering his lungs. Pierre Robin sequence was diagnosed and his mother obtained a book which described how best to feed a child with this syndrome. Against all the odds Tim recovered from this poor start in life, and began to thrive.

His parents soon realised that his elbow and knee joints were enlarged and his fingers stiff. He appeared also to be very hard of

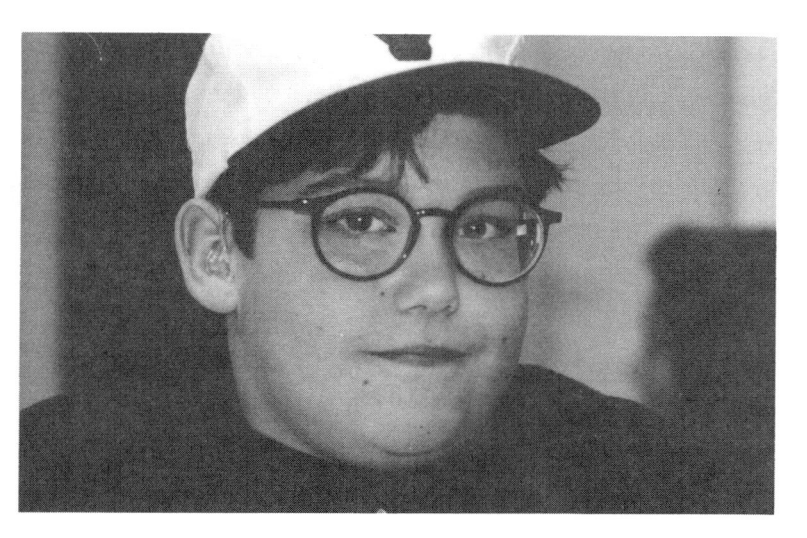

Tim Weisselberger

hearing. Despite these difficulties he was a happy, lovable child which made it easier for his parents to cope. When I first met him I was immediately struck by his wonderful sense of humour and cheerfulness which, despite the language barrier, came across loud and clear.

When Tim started to walk he moved about with a very unsure gait, almost like a penguin, and had periods of severe pain in his knees, hips and feet. On many days he couldn't move at all. When the doctors were told this, they said that he had probably fallen in the playground and would get over it.

At the age of three Tim was fitted with two hearing aids to help him communicate more easily with his playmates. He attended an ordinary kindergarten, albeit with help once a week from a speech therapist and a teacher from the School for the Deaf. Despite continually suffering colds, ear infections, aching joints and high fevers, Tim's life was bearable. That is, until one day, when picking him up from school, his mother found Tim's teacher staring in disbelief at his right eye. A large white spot had appeared in the centre of the eye, almost covering the pupil. His mother immediately took him to the GP who was unable to help but arranged for a specialist to see Tim within a week. The consultant was amazed to find that, at the age of five, Tim had a 'ripe' cataract, something she had never seen in a child so young. Because of inexperience, she felt unable to help but made an appointment for him to be seen at the

Amsterdam Medical Centre - one of the largest university hospitals in the Netherlands. The doctors confirmed that Tim needed an operation within a month if he was to retain any useful sight. His mother was told to ring admissions for them to arrange a date for the operation. She said she rang the number so many times they became fed up with her. However, 29 days after seeing the specialist Tim was operated on successfully. As Tim was very myopic and too young to have a lens implant a contact lens and a pair of glasses were prescribed.

His parents asked if there was any connection between all his symptoms, but the consultants said it was purely coincidental. The eye problem probably was caused by a blow, although Tim was equally adamant that he had not been hit.

Thankfully, fate was on Tim's side. One day, during a routine visit to the hospital, an eye specialist said she felt the problems were connected by some unknown common cause such as a metabolic disorder. After a series of tests, Tim was referred to a Genetic Centre where at the age of eight Stickler syndrome at last was diagnosed. Tests were carried out on the family and Tim's father was found to have the condition, although in a much milder form. For him, childhood difficulties were finally made clear and an unexplained back pain understood.

The doctors told Tim's mother that no one else in The Netherlands was affected by the condition nor could anyone advise her about it.

Desperate to know more she began her search for information. This quest finally led her to Dr Passarge at the University in Essen, Germany, and then to Dr Stickler in America. Both were extremely helpful, and when Dr Stickler travelled to Germany for a guest tutorial at the Medical school at Essen University, he asked Dr Passarge to invite Tim along to meet him.

For a number of years Tim and his mother travelled to Essen to appear before geneticists, paediatricians and Gps. His mother would tell the story about her battle to find a diagnosis for her son and ended by showing photographs of Tim with the distinctive features of a 'Stickler' baby. In exchange the medical students would examine Tim, ask questions about the condition and how they both coped with its everyday problems. His mother also re-enforced her claim that the medical profession in general should listen to parents and patients who, although not medically trained, can give vital clues to aid diagnosis. These visits, with the usual round of applause, a gift of a toy and lunch in the University's restaurant were once enjoyed but now that he is older, Tim no longer goes to Essen. Instead, his mother keeps in contact with Dr Passarge by letter, sending him photographs of Tim and diagrams of surgery carried out.

Since Tim's diagnosis, his mother has contacted several Stickler syndrome families in The Netherlands and Belgium. She translates medical reports into Dutch so that these families have a better insight into the condition and is immersed in answering questions, reassuring parents, and putting families with similar problems in touch with one another. When I last visited her she was pleased that at last doctors were beginning to recognise Stickler Syndrome. I asked her if she had any advice to offer a parent with a 'Stickler' child. She said 'Enjoy life to the full. Don't be over-protective, ensure the child has a wide range of interests to occupy time and encourage the child to have lots of friends'.

In the short time I have known Tim he has undergone many joint operations and remained cheerful, but respiratory problems are now a constant worry. Although Tim's father has been relatively symptom free until now, he has recently begun to experience severe joint problems and is now awaiting surgery on his spine.

MELICA:

Melica studied medicine at Southampton Medical School, an interest resulting from her many visits to hospitals as a child. She was one of four children, two of whom died soon after birth. Melica was born with a cleft palate, a small hole in the heart, a squint and is very short-sighted. The heart problem is not, as far as we know, related to Stickler syndrome. She was diagnosed as having Pierre-Robin sequence.

Melica says she was never good at sports, so favoured subjects like maths and the sciences and has fond memories of the music department. She played the piano from the age of seven, and at 13 took up the clarinet, her favourite instrument. A highlight in her life came in 1986 when her concert band won the school band section of the National Festival of Music for Youth, and she played in the school proms at the Royal Albert Hall in London.

Her mother recalls that Stickler syndrome was not diagnosed, but in passing it was briefly mentioned when Melica's brother was admitted to Bristol Eye Hospital with a detached retina three years ago. Sadly, this was diagnosed too late and her brother is now blind in one eye.

In September 1990, through her medical studies, she met Dr Karen Temple of Southampton General Hospital and Stickler syndrome was finally diagnosed.

Melica qualified as a doctor in 1994, having also obtained a B.Sc degree in psychology during her time at Southampton University.

She intends to pursue a career in either general practise or psychiatry and hopes to treat her future patients as people, not a collection of signs and symptoms. As she says, she knows what it is like to feel up against a brick wall and wants to treat her patients with the understanding and respect she expects for herself.

STEPHANIE AND LOUISE:

Another family from the Southampton area, the Uphills, have two children affected by Stickler syndrome. Stephanie, the second child, was born in January 1987 and I have outlined her case in Chapter Six.

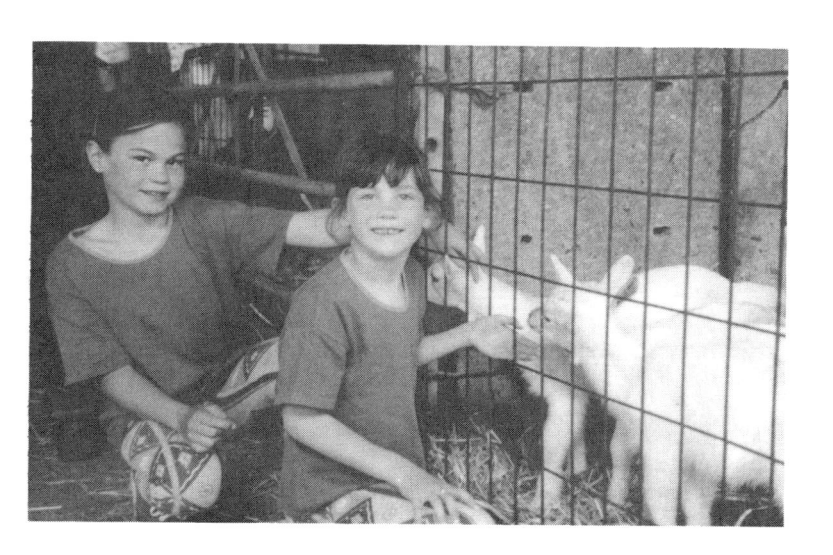

Stephanie and Louise Uphill

After Stephanie was born, the local authorities were good and organised a home help for a few hours each week until she was a year old.

Stephanie started play-group and, although she slept well, she ate irregularly. Her mother was concerned that the disorder could be passed on, and when Stephanie was two and a half, asked her GP to refer her to the Genetics Department of the Southampton General Hospital. After investigating the family background it was concluded that Stephanie had Stickler syndrome, and not Pierre Robin sequence. Furthermore, Louise, her elder sister, was also diagnosed. The condition was passed to both girls by their father, Stephen.

As a child Stephen had suffered badly with pain in the hips and had been diagnosed as suffering from a disorder in which the top surface of the joint deteriorates. This causes decalcification, the fluid of the joint crystallises and pain is caused during movement. Further investigation found that Stickler syndrome was passed to Stephen from his father who had suffered from 'rheumatism' from an early age, had 'bad' ears, poor vision as well as a cleft palate. Another member of Stephen's family has arthritic involvement of the fingers and ankles, both being deformed, and several years ago underwent surgery for detached retinas. She also has a typically flat face with no nasal bridge. Yet another member of the family was born with no palate at all and investigations have revealed that Stephen's paternal grandmother had extremely poor vision, wore very thick glasses and had arthritis of the spine. When photographs were shown to the geneticist she confirmed the grandmother had a typical Stickler syndrome face.

Stephanie is now six years old and has been at school a year. She enjoys joining in games, learning to read and write, and misbehaving when the mood takes her - in fact everything you would expect from a normal happy child of this age.

Her sister Louise shows no outward signs of the condition, the only indication being a very slight cleft in her uvula. Both girls are affected adversely by food colouring allergies - a common disorder in children.

KIRSTY AND LOUISE:

The Fisher family, from Surrey, are another family that knows only too well the distress and irritation that Stickler syndrome can bring. When Angela was expecting her first baby in 1983 she was so excited, especially as she had experienced a miscarriage a year earlier. However, the due date came and went, and the doctors decided she should be induced. A few painful hours followed and finally Kirsty arrived, but the feelings of euphoria very quickly turned to fear. It was obvious, even to a new mum that something was seriously wrong. Kirsty had the biggest eyes Angela had ever seen, and her little face appeared to be flat, but the main concern was the baby's breathing. Angela had never heard such an erratic and laboured noise before.

Kirsty was whisked away to the special care unit and her parents did not see her again for almost 24 hours. In the early days a nurse came to see her and explained that Kirsty was to be transferred to Great Ormond Street Hospital in London because of her poor health. However, it was later decided that she should remain at the Guildford Hospital where she had been born and arrangements were made for her paediatrician to remain in constant contact with Great Ormond Street by fax. The paediatrician turned out to be a tower of strength to the family. He explained that Kirsty had a cleft of the soft palate and that was causing her breathing problems. He confirmed also that she had an underdeveloped chin, and was possibly suffering from Pierre Robin sequence. Like many other families this was later re-diagnosed as Stickler syndrome, and further investigation revealed that Kirsty had inherited the condition from her father.

Meanwhile, Kirsty was placed in an incubator and given oxygen. She was also tube fed and given medication through her open tummy button. She also had a naso-pharyngeal tube inserted into her nose and down her throat. This tube was to prevent Kirsty's tongue obstructing the airway. The tube was held in place by sticking plaster and medical sellotape and when Angela next saw her baby all she could see of her face was her mouth and eyes - the rest was completely covered in plaster. The memories of the shock of seeing such a small baby in this way is still with Angela today.

Kirsty remained in this state for two weeks before the plaster and

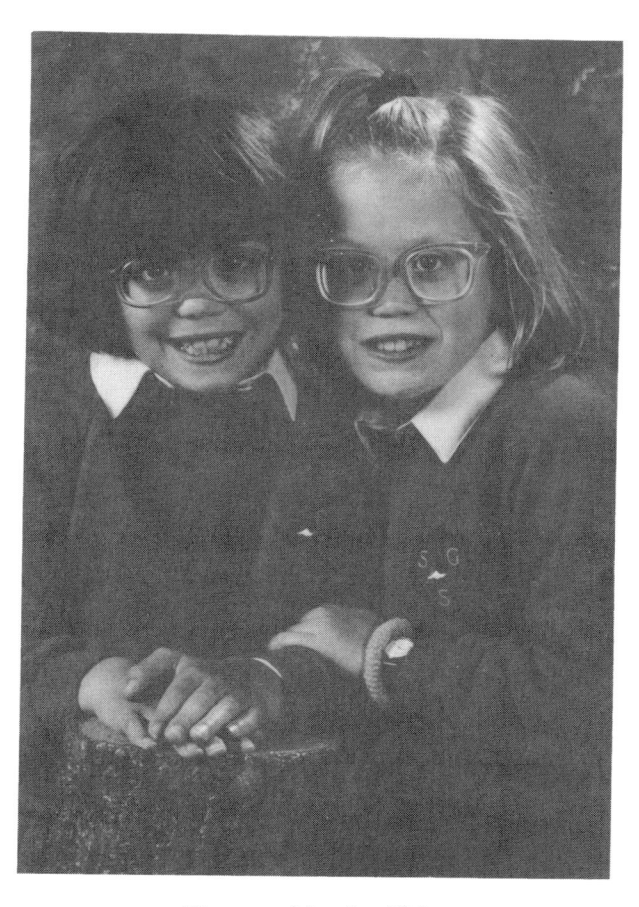

Kirsty and Louise Fisher

tube were removed to see if she could breathe without her tongue falling back and blocking her airway. Angela was so excited. She longed to hold her baby and gaze into her face. However the elation soon turned to shock when Angela saw that Kirsty's face was blotchy and sore owing to the plaster, and that it looked even flatter than she remembered. However the shock passed and Angela arranged for her parents to see their grandchild for the first time. They arrived at the Special Care Baby Unit to be told that there had been a major setback. Kirsty hadn't been able to control her tongue and it had fallen back over the airway and she could not breathe. They watched, in shocked horror, as the specialist came dashing down the corridor to try and save her. The family were rushed out of the unit into a waiting room to await news. 'I was absolutely devastated,' said Angela. 'I thought little Kirsty would die, and if she did manage to survive, she would be brain damaged.'

The minutes ticked by, each one feeling as though it was an hour, until eventually the doctor came and told them that they had managed, after a struggle, to re-insert the naso-pharyngeal tube, and that Kirsty's vital signs were returning to normal.

Kirsty stayed in hospital for six weeks from her birth with the tube inserted for much of that time. Angela was eventually able to bring her home for, firstly, an afternoon, then overnight, then a weekend and finally for good. But baby arrived home with an array of equipment - oxygen, an aprioea blanket to monitor her breathing at night and a pack containing everything needed to insert a nasopharyngeal tube. Wherever Kirsty went the pack went with her, and did so until she was fifteen months old.

Kirsty is now eleven and half years old. She wears two hearing aids and has severe myopia. She has had two operations on her palate - one the repair and the second, to improve her speech. Until she was seven, Kirsty also suffered febrile convulsions, most worrying for the family, because of the fear that her tongue would obstruct the airway and stop her from breathing. This happened only once, at a birthday party, when the emergency services had to be called to resuscitate her!

Kirsty is able to attend a normal school and has extra help to ensure that she has understood the class work. Small print textbooks are enlarged for her, as are maps etc. She also wears a radio microphone so that she is able to hear the teacher clearly. Today she is a happy well adjusted youngster and her mother is extremely proud of her.

Seventeen months after Kirsty's birth her sister Louise arrived on Valentine's Day 1985. In the run up to her birth, and because the specialists now knew about Stickler syndrome, Angela had countless scans. After one of these scans in the sixth month of pregnancy the hospital thought that they could detect a definite cleft in the unborn baby's palate. This left Angela with three months in which to come to terms with the fact that she was likely to have to go through all the stress and problems for a second time.

However, when Louise was born there was no cleft in the palate! The hospital had got it wrong. Far from feeling euphoric, as everyone had anticipated, Angela felt confused and unable to accept her new baby. She was convinced that something would go wrong. Louise did indeed have the same facial features as Kirsty, but her nose was 'button' and not totally flat. The doctors did their best to reassure Angela but to no avail. Unfortunately Angela could not come to terms with the fact that her new baby was able to be with her all the time. Louise spent the night of her birth in the Special Care Baby Unit, and everyone hoped that a good night's sleep would help her mother to come to terms with the situation. However, the next afternoon Angela went down to see Louise in the Baby Unit only to find her looking extremely ill. Her colour was ashen and she appeared to be struggling for breath. The paediatrician was called and diagnosed fluid on the lungs. Louise was put onto a drip and remained in hospital for a week. Strangely, after this incident, Angela felt relieved and to this day cannot explain why!

Despite her problems, Louise progressed very well. It was discovered that she was myopic and had impaired hearing, but not to the same degree as her sister. However, she also suffered febrile convulsions which were more of a worry for her mother than any one else.

Louise is now 10 years old, and a very striking girl with olive skin and gorgeous dark hair. She wears glasses, needs two hearing aids, and has flat feet and wears inserts in her shoes. Her school work is excellent and she is an extremely happy, intelligent girl.

But although Angela has two girls to be extremely proud of, unfortunately, the strain of hospital appointments, visits to the doctors, emergencies, and numerous school visits to explain the condition have sadly taken its toll.

Angela's marriage failed and, although Stickler syndrome was not the reason, it was a major contributing factor. She feels that she should have been stronger at the time and battled on, but in the end she was mentally and physically exhausted.

However Angela's story does have a happy ending. She is now married again with two more children - a girl called Rosie and a boy called Jack - both perfectly healthy. All of the children get on extremely well and Rosie is becoming quite an expert on Stickler syndrome, despite her tender age of five.

Angela says, 'Discovering Stickler syndrome has changed my life dramatically. I have had to learn to cope with things that I would never have done if Stickler syndrome hadn't entered my life. Stickler syndrome is a pain and a nuisance, but we live with it and I think that our lives have been made richer because of it'. Her advice to newly diagnosed parents, 'Don't lose heart, Stickler syndrome is not the end of the world, just the beginning of a different one.'

CHAPTER NINE

COPING WITH A CHILD AFFECTED BY STICKLER SYNDROME

Birth should be a joyful experience for every parent, but sadly, for many families it is marred by the arrival of a child with a genetic disorder.

For some it is the first time that they are aware of the condition; for others it brings confirmation of their worst fears. Depending on the severity, it can present the family with problems and challenges that continue throughout life, and helping children to achieve their full potential and development may feel like an enormous burden.

Although it is the parents who have to face the daily problems and maintain a level of progress, they should *not* bear the responsibility alone. The parents' instinctive feelings about their child were not always recognised in the past, but thankfully today, more parents are being asked to contribute their ideas at consultations and their observations are noted and regarded with respect.

As mentioned elsewhere, it is vital that anyone suffering from an inherited disorder like Stickler syndrome, or anyone who is a member of a family where someone has been born with a genetic disorder, should be given specialist genetic counselling. It is vital too that the information given to families, either to the parents or related members, is fully understood. Still reeling from the shock, it is only natural that some people cannot comprehend what is being said. Many questions will surface - why us, what have we done, how will I cope, what about the future? Families must realise that prevention is in their hands, and although this can be heart-breaking news, at least families will be aware of the possible consequences of having another child. Some 8% of all children born have a genetic problem, but only a fraction of these have a serious or life-threatening condition. Many, like families affected by Stickler syndrome, have a whole range of disabilities ranging from very mild to very severe, and each should be assessed individually. It is only then that the best treatments and help can be sought and obtained.

Families, especially parents, should in no way blame themselves, yet the feelings of guilt, the responsibility, and a sense of failure can be overwhelming. Both parents, and often both sets of grandparents may need careful counselling, especially if the child is severely affected in one or more of the features of the condition. Many families benefit from the shared experience of family discussions, especially at times of surgery. Organisations such as the Stickler Syndrome Support Group can help to reassure parents. Look, The National Federation of Families with Visually Impaired Children, can provide support and education advice concerning a visually impaired child. CLAPA - The Cleft Lip and Palate Association can help with problems relating to feeding problems. GIG - the Genetic Interest Group can help with genetic queries. The addresses for these and other organisations are included in the *'Useful Organisations and Addresses'* section.

Although those born with the Pierre-Robin anomalies have feeding difficulties which can be distressing, these children often fair much better, because they require the services of a Special Care Baby Unit with a dedicated team of paediatricians who monitor and look after their progress. Such children at least have the advantage of being properly assessed, especially if Stickler syndrome is known to be within that family unit. Each is quickly diagnosed. Remember, it is thanks to a caring paediatrician that this disorder was defined. Accurate and early diagnosis is vital for any child with disabilities.

Babies born with a visual impairment will be referred to a specialist very quickly, but the parents themselves must form part of the team which considers the child's welfare. No one sees the child more than the parents, and they may be the first people to be aware that something is amiss. Their observations are invaluable.

Whether a child is born with visual defects or acquires them later, the news is always devastating. Blindness seems to instill more fear for parents, family and friends than any other disability, and until quite recently visual impairment made everyone feel inadequate and an object of pity. Anyone who still has these feelings should visit a blind school for a day and watch children without sight running around and playing confidently out of doors. It is a most uplifting and rewarding experience.

People generally do not appreciate how severely deafness can handicap a child, or understand that speech and communication depend upon hearing. Therefore early diagnosis of a hearing loss is vital, and it is rare today to find a child over the age of two who is undiagnosed, although sadly it can happen. There are statutory obligations for health visitors to examine a baby's hearing at eight months. However if a parent suspects a problem, an earlier referral should be requested. By eight months a baby already may have lost valuable hearing skills, and many families say that their child's problems would have been far less traumatic if only they could have been diagnosed sooner. Sensorineural deafness is a difficult condition to diagnose and cannot be corrected. The degree of damage varies from a mild to a complete loss of hearing. As mentioned previously, another problem associated with Stickler syndrome is otitis media, or glue ear.

Children who suffer from hearing difficulties miss a great deal of what is going on around them and in the classroom, and consequently standards fall below those of other pupils. They flounder, trying to comprehend what it is that other children find so easy, and their school work and social development can be seriously affected. Deafness needs proper assessment at an audiological centre, so that corrective measures can be taken quickly, and the management of the child's disability discussed. In this way the potential loss of language communication and comprehension will be reduced.

The age at which a child begins to speak varies a great deal, and often parents become anxious if there appears to be a delay. If it is established that the child hears clear tones, then there is no cause for alarm. However, if a hearing loss is discovered and a hearing aid is recommended it should be serviced regularly, and the batteries checked daily. It can be very worrying for a young child to be suddenly flung into a world of muffled tones when a battery needs changing. Loop circuit systems in classrooms and radiophone aids are available so that teachers at school and parents at home can stay in touch with a deaf child without having to be very close.

If there are any real speech problems, or cleft palate or other oral surgery carried out, the child will need to see a speech therapist. The number who work solely with children has reduced drastically in recent years, and is now considered to be below an acceptable level. Even if this were not the case, no professional could possibly give enough time to an individual child to enable him or her to reach his or her full potential. However, parents have more resources and useful knowledge within·themselves than they ever take credit for. Parents sometimes shy away from helping, fearing they are useless, but they will soon realise that they can do a great deal to help their child. A speech therapist can teach them how to put that knowledge to good use so that their child can obtain the maximum help. Parents should learn to speak clearly, preferably facing the child and encourage others to do the same. Pictures can be read and used for describing activities to a child. Enlarging screens make it possible for a child with poor vision to read books, and there are a number of braille printing devices which enable a child to join in classes by producing his or her own material. Radio and television is no substitute for personal attention, especially when the child has a visual impairment too.

Children with multiple handicaps find one disability hampers their progress in overcoming another, or even creates other problems. Loss of vision can mean there is a delayed mobility because a child who cannot see clearly has no desire to get up and explore. Similarly a child with aching joints may not want to crawl or run around and explore the 'seeing world' Loss of hearing means loss of speech development which in turn leads to frustration and could result in behaviour problems.

Coming to terms with multiple disability, and accepting whatever that may entail, is essential for all concerned. Parents can read about Stickler syndrome, talk to others with the disorder and read books in general concerning disability and learning difficulties. There is a list of books at the back of this book, but seek out others. Local libraries, health visitors or social workers will help if asked.

It is not always possible to forecast what the future will hold, so the best solution is to seek out those aspects of a child which are normal, and work on what the child can do really well. We all have hidden talents and it is up to a parent to try and discover a child's hidden potential. Families need time to become accustomed to the idea of multiple disability, and they must have some positive factors to encourage them to cope better.

In an ideal world, any child, handicapped or not, should be accepted into a community, but sadly we do not live in an ideal world. Attitudes are slowly changing, but not quick enough. Some people are so ignorant of handicap and have so little understanding that they are downright cruel - knowingly or unknowingly. Every handicapped child is cherished by the family, but not always by others. Parents are often hurt by comments like: 'That ought to be put down,' or 'Poor little thing, what sort of a life will it have?' When this happens, and it will, parents will feel shocked and angry; it may even reduce them to tears, but after a time they will get used to it. There is no point in telling someone with such an attitude that the child is loved, has great potential, or is artistic or capable of doing senior school maths in junior school. It is best to smile and inwardly think of all the excellent progress a child has already made.

Able-bodied children accept others with disabilities far better than adults and perhaps it is time we learnt the art of acceptance from them. The integration of those affected by Stickler syndrome into society is the way forward, but until people became educated to understand disability, there must be ample support and advice.

A number of benefits are available to help with the financial burden of coping with a handicapped child, and parents need to know what can be claimed and at what age. They will also need to know what other relevant criteria needs to be detailed to make a claim. Rules and regulations change frequently, and health visitors or social workers can help, or a local Benefits Agency. Also, the local Citizens Advice Bureau is a useful source of information, as is the local library. Families who have children with special needs will find that social workers will give practical and sympathetic advice. Part of their job is to ensure the well-being of all children in their area, at all times. They will also know about special local services, local charities that may be able to help, and make recommendations for holidays and respite care. This is a vital lifeline for the well being of both parents and child.

Education begins in the cradle and parents should never underestimate their own value and ability to instill in their children an interest and a love for learning. For children affected by Stickler syndrome, things may not be so easy. A child who cannot hear or does not see too well, or who cannot crawl or run quickly is disadvantaged. But whatever the degree of disability a child is entitled to a good education, an acceptable quality of life, and equal opportunities for success.

Pre-school education is important for slow developers to enable them to reach an average standard by the time they reach school age. Some areas provide a service whereby a visiting teacher will call weekly to teach the child at home. Check availability with a Social worker.

Local education authorities are required to give the fullest co-operation to parents seeking information about schools in their area, and parents often feel a great responsibility when they come to choose a school for a child with any disability, however mild. The choice may depend upon a number of factors such as the area, facilities and the school's reputation. If the child has a friend in that school, it is certainly an advantage. But parents should make sure that the school is within a reasonable distance and has easy access, especially if the child is confined to a wheelchair or has visual impairment. Before a child starts school it may be helpful to staff to know a little about Stickler syndrome. A variety of literature can be obtained from the Stickler Syndrome Support Group, and a leaflet - Stickler Syndrome - What is it? is available to anyone on request.

Today children with special needs can be catered for within their own localities and this helps them to became accepted members of their communities. The future needs of the child have to be planned, and a regular meeting, attended by all those who are involved with the child, including the parents', should be sought whenever the immediate and long term plans are to be discussed.

PARENTS' QUESTIONS ANSWERED

How can I tell if my young baby is visually impaired?

Parents may find that their baby does not reach to play with mobile toys, their toes, or look towards people nearby. If you suspect that your baby is visually impaired, contact your health visitor or GP immediately. The general development of children with visual impairment calls for specialised training, and individual assessment is vital.

How can I stimulate a child with poor vision or no vision at all?

You may think it is difficult to stimulate a child who is already disadvantaged by visual impairment, but with a little thought it can turn into a rewarding experience for both the child and the parent. Very few children are without some degree of vision, but you must always be awake to the possibility of stimulating any residual vision, helping them to use what they have to the best advantage. A child will sense if you are nervous, so have faith in yourself and do not hesitate. Have fun and enjoy the experience of learning together.

There are numerous ways to stimulate a baby. The following are some examples but do not be afraid to try out your own ideas.

1. Sew bells onto pieces of ribbon or elastic and attach to your

baby's wrists and ankles. This will help baby to relate to movements.

2. Play different types of music and see to which type of music the baby best responds.
3. Wear brightly coloured clothes so that the baby can see you, and exaggerate all movements.
4. Wear the same perfume everyday so that baby can identify with you.
5. Always say when you are entering or leaving a room. Talk as you approach a baby, especially if you are going to touch him or her. Sudden movement can cause fright.
6. Show baby brightly coloured toys and always remember that the light should be behind or at the side of the child.
7. Talk to baby all the time. Tell him or her what you are doing or where you are going.
8. Never say 'it,' always name the object and say things like round ball or square tin, soft toy or hard book.
9. Put baby on a furry or long piled rug. Tiny fingers can grasp the shag as they roll over, and it helps them to feel safe.
10. Take baby outside often and tell him\her what makes a sound or produces a certain smell. Be aware of all the senses, and use them to full advantage.
11. Contact the Occupational or Speech Therapist as they can give advice on movement, feeding and adapting adapt your home.

12. As the child grows remember to leave doors completely open or completely closed, so there is no danger of the child walking into them.

Who should I contact when I know my child is visually impaired?

As soon as it is realised that a child has a visual impairment a 'VI Peri', or Advisory/Peripatetic Teacher for the Visually Impaired should be contacted. This person,(in some authorities there are several), is a qualified teacher of the visually impaired who will travel around schools and homes. If your child also has a hearing problem you may be told of the Sensory Impairment Service too. The help and advice of a VI Peri teacher is essential and can make a huge difference to a child's early development.

How much support can I expect regarding my child's education?

The amount of support a child needs will depend upon the severity of the impairment. If the child needs substantial resources, in both time and equipment, the VI peri teacher or the child's school may make a request for an assessment of the child's needs, but a parent may do so by writing to a Statementing Officer. This is a person who is responsible for the statementing process, and they are usually based in a Special Needs section of the local Education Department or at the Area Education Offices.

Although the Statementing Officer is responsible for writing the Statement, the assessment is based upon a report supplied. Often the child is represented by an Educational psychologist who will provide a report on the child's social skills and collect evidence of strengths and weaknesses. Before the final assessment report can be completed, a report from a qualified VI teacher, the educational psychologist and a consultant ophthalmologist should be obtained. A parent will also be asked to make a contribution to the report, and this is very important. A parent may also wish other professionals who are involved in the child's need to contribute their findings and these should be sent as part of the parent's contribution.

CHAPTER TEN

HELPING YOURSELF TO A BETTER WAY OF LIFE

This chapter is for young people and adults affected by Stickler syndrome. It aims to help them approach life in a more positive way, and offers help and advice to enable them to cope. Most of the advice in this chapter is included in the question and answer format and is based on the most frequently questions asked.

Remember, if a particular need is not mentioned, ask the professionals for advice or contact the Stickler Syndrome Support Group, who may be able to put you in touch with the appropriate authority or organisation. If you don't get a satisfactory reply, then keep on asking until you do. It may sound selfish, but you are the most important person in this situation, and you are entitled to a better way of life. Living with Stickler syndrome can be difficult enough without making it harder on yourself. Be positive.

Once Stickler syndrome has been diagnosed, the genetic implications fully explained, and the correct programme of treatment begun, you should be thinking about the future. The prime concern is to achieve and maintain a level of life that is acceptable to you, and only you will know what makes life satisfactory.

It is important to realise that an affected person is going to be faced with some limitations throughout life. These will range from comparatively minor difficulties such as not being able to see clearly, knocking over the odd glass, or suffering from painful joints, to needing someone physically to take you out and about, and the possible trauma of major surgery. It may even mean a change of career, which, although worrying at the time, could end up as a rewarding and exciting experience.

The most important point to bear in mind is that you should *never* give in to difficulties. With a little thought, there is always a way around everything.

Any affected person should be encouraged to live life to the full, although leisure activities involving vigorous exertion or lifting should be avoided. Try to be as independent as possible without turning into a martyr. No one will thank you for struggling, so make it easier for yourself. I still manage to travel alone. I take a taxi to my nearest railway station, and can go alone to familiar places. If I am going to a function in an unfamiliar place with friends, I arrange to meet them at the railway station and we go together. People are only too willing to help if you ask. They may not offer because they don't want to offend or embarrass you, or may simply overlook your problem. There have been many times, especially at night when my vision is almost nil, when a friend has dashed across the road, leaving me standing on the other side, or walked out of a building, forgetting that I will need a guiding arm. In some ways it is pleasant when this happens, as it makes me feel that I am at least 'normal' to those who are closest to me.

If you are visually impaired then PLEASE use a symbol or long cane at all times. Without one, it is no good complaining when someone knocks into you, or even worse, when you are knocked down by a car.

Operations can be numerous for those affected by Stickler syndrome, but being in contact with someone who has been through a similar experience can help. Support from family and friends is important too. Speak freely about your condition and your worries about pending treatment or surgery. Make sure you are aware of what is going to happen, why a certain operation is being performed and how long you can expect to be incapacitated. Knowing all the facts will help to overcome the feeling of isolation.

Obviously you are going to get your 'down' days, but try to keep busy and have plenty of interests. Try not to think of the long term future either. Live each day as it comes. My writing has carried me through many a 'down' day, and I believe I would not have coped with my many operations if I had not had my writing to occupy my mind. If you allow yourself to be miserable, friends will swiftly get fed up, cease to visit, and forget to invite you out. Soon you will find that life has turned into a downward spiral.

Today, with the help of various organisations and support services, there is no need for anyone with difficulties to feel isolated, and there is nothing that cannot be achieved. It may mean that you have to look for a slightly different way of doing things, but if you accept this as a sort of competition that you MUST win, then you will find that life takes on a whole new dimension. Set yourself targets and aim to achieve them, but don't get too dispirited if you cannot reach your goals. What does success mean to you? For the able-bodied it may mean sailing around the world, but for someone affected by Stickler syndrome it may mean a short walk to the shops, or getting to the end of the day without giving in to joint pain. Whenever you aims, when you do achieve something, feel proud and reward yourself!

Never try to fight your battles alone. There is a big difference between accepting help, and giving in and allowing others to take over your life. We all need help. You cannot do it alone. Wellington, the Iron Duke, had an army, so did Cromwell, so call upon your own personal army of family, friends and back-up services. They are there to help and support you.

There is a mountain of help out there. Unfortunately, our needs are so individual, and only you can make them known in the right areas, thus enabling yourself to benefit from all the available help.

To sum up, living with Stickler syndrome can be frustrating and downright annoying. It can reduce you to tears, but when things go well it can also be rewarding. Your life will be a mixture of set backs and great achievements, but then, so are the lives of most people. How you cope with the condition is entirely up to you, and I hope this book has helped you to put your hopes and fears into perspective. There is plenty of help in the world, but we MUST help ourselves too. Perseverance, a determination to succeed at all costs, and total acceptance of a situation that is beyond our control are the prime factors to consider.

Admittedly, living with the condition can be hard, but the gift of life is the most precious asset we have, so enjoy it. This is not a life threatening condition, so be positive, be happy. Live each day as it comes, learn to appreciate the simpler things in life, and life will reward you with all her bounty. The world is your oyster - IT IS UP TO YOU TO MAKE THE MOST OF YOUR LIFE.

YOUR QUESTIONS ON A BETTER WAY OF LIFE ANSWERED

I love gardening, but find it difficult to bend. How can I overcome this problem?

This is a common problem, but it can be overcome by building your garden up to waist height. Walls made of ordinary slabs can be filled with rubble before applying a good thick layer of garden soil. Flowers and vegetables can be separated, and will make planting and weeding easy. A raised garden can be the ideal solution for wheelchair users too.

Any advice on help with failing sight?

Failing eyesight is the most devastating feature of this condition, and if the sufferer has to give up work as well, the trauma will be even greater. It is essential that the person concerned is encouraged to lead a new, meaningful life.

If you are registered as partially sighted, and are still able to work, then your first visit should be to the local Disability Employment Officer who can help with retraining, or suggest aids to help to enable you to carry on with your job or start a new career. Your assigned Rehabilitation Officer will be able to advise you on what is on offer in your own area.

If you are medically retired, then I cannot stress too much the importance of finding an absorbing hobby or interest. Although your skills may be limited, there may be some local charity that you could help. Involve the family. Tell them you want to find some new interests and enlist their help in finding something suitable. Perhaps there is something that you have always wanted to pursue, but never had the time before. Now is the time! A newly acquired talent could possibly lead to a career in another field.

Don't forget your local Adult Education Centres. Most offer a substantial discount for disabled students. Besides the usual batch of academic subjects there is usually a programme of leisure activities, as well as a series of 'one off' lectures, even 'Saturday schools'. Seven years ago, with time on my hands, I enrolled for a Creative Writing Course and joined a non-academic course on the History of Medicine. Over the past few years I have studied the development of medicine from the 15th century to the 19th century, and have learnt a great deal about the attitudes of the times. These courses have also given me a greater insight into the struggles of our ancestors, and I have come to appreciate the skills of the surgeons of today. It is not too long ago that the surgeon had to amputate without anaesthesia, and there are many tales of surgeons being physically sick before an operation, knowing the pain they were about to inflict on their wretched patients. I have also learned a great deal about social history and how war has helped to equip surgeons with many skills they perhaps would never have achieved otherwise. For the less squeamish there are courses in art appreciation, flower arranging, pottery, bridge, etc.

My vision has deteriorated, can I be registered, and if so, what are the benefits?

If vision deteriorates to a degree that the patient needs to be registered as partially sighted, or as 'technically' blind, you should talk this over with your ophthalmic surgeon, who will need to fill in a BD8 form. This certifies that the person's sight is sufficiently poor to warrant registration.

Registration should never be considered the end. It is just the beginning of another way of life. When I was registered as partially sighted, my main concern was that I might have to give up writing. Not so. My Rehabilitation Officer suggested a visit to my local resource centre for the visually impaired, where I was shown a collection of magnifiers, lighting, and even binocular spectacles that could help me, even a software enlarge facility for my word processor.

What can a local Resource centre offer?

Most counties have a Resource Centre for the visually impaired, and your Rehabilitation Officer will be very keen for you to visit it as soon as possible. There you will find a variety of aids to help you around the home and with leisure activities. Make sure you tell your

Rehabilitation Officer all about yourself - your interest, what you enjoy doing most, and more importantly what you miss doing. These centres also run a variety of courses for things like microwave cookery, coping about the house, computer technology, craft, and braille lessons for those who need them.

I have just completed a six week rehabilitation course at my local resource centre and I must say that although I was apprehensive about attending, it proved to be most beneficial and enabled me to try out things I would have thought impossible with failing sight. The mornings were spent in the kitchen and we were all encouraged to try out new methods of coping with cooking etc. After preparing, cooking and eating a two course lunch the afternoons were taken up with a variety of interesting topics including coming to terms with failing sight, gardening, relaxation and applying make-up for the visually impaired. I finished the course with more confidence and a sense of achievement.

Is there anywhere else that I can obtain help and advice?
The RNIB have a wealth of information and advice to help blind and partially sighted people, and a telephone call to their Peterborough office, details in *'Useful Organisations and Addresses'* will bring you an information pack, outlining all they have to offer. Also available free of charge are print, braille and cassette copies of its aims and strategy entitled *Meeting the Needs of Visually Handicapped People*.

Also the Partially Sighted Society provides equipment and offers advice on all aspects of living or working with a visual impairment. Details of membership and an application form are available on request. Address in *'Useful Organisations and addresses'* section.

Anyone with a visual loss should consider buying a copying of the IN TOUCH Handbook. This is an annual publication published by the BBC Radio 4 Broadcasting Support Services and is an excellent guide for people with a visual handicap.

Any advice about adjusting my home?

Think about your home as it is now and be prepared to make a few minor adjustments. For example, if your working surfaces are white, then don't use white plates. Think of colour co-ordination all the time. Glassware is invisible to a person with failing sight, so use a patterned, smoked or coloured glass. Experiment with colours, depending on your visual loss, some are more distinctive than others. Similarly, never cook mince in a brown dish.

I find it very difficult to distinguish between black and navy, so keep my navy belt on a navy skirt and the black one on a black skirt. Devise a system where all black shoes are kept in a box or plastic bag and all navy ones are left without a cover. Men can keep a co-ordinated tie around the neck of a shirt or hang whole outfits - jackets and trousers that match should be hung together. There is nothing more frustrating than dressing for an appointment, only to find that you are uncertain of the colour of the garment you want to wear. With a little thought beforehand you can become quite independent.

It is a case of learning new skills to compensate for poor vision. The RNIB distributes colour indicating buttons in 16 different shapes, each one representing a different colour. For example red is represented by a cross, green a shamrock and blue by a star. These can be sewn into the seam of a garment if vision cannot distinguish colours.

I have to rely on other people to read my letters and it depresses to me to think I cannot read them myself.

This can be very frustrating, and if you cannot manage with a magnifier, then you may like to consider the possibility of purchasing an 'EEZEE Reader'. This takes the form of a lightweight hand held scanner, which can be tuned to a spare channel on your television set. The scanner is placed on the material to be read and the words appear, greatly magnified in black and white on your TV screen. It is expensive, but may be a worthwhile investment if you have to rely on other people more than you wish. Again, details of the reader can be found in the *'Useful Organisations and Addresses'* section.

I am finding it difficult to do the leisure activities I once enjoyed. Any tips on how to deal with this?

As the majority of Stickler patients in adult life experience difficulty with sight and have joint problems, leisure interests of a sporting type may be difficult or impossible. It is very important, therefore, to find a new or existing interest you are able to pursue within your limitations. This not only gives you something to do, but also keeps your mind occupied, and will help prevent depression.

Make life easy for yourself by accepting offers of lifts and a guiding arm where necessary. I have found that people are only too willing to help if you make your needs known. In fact, diplomacy is the name of the game with the many offers of a lift I receive to college. Some people, however, back away for fear of offending, so it is up to us to meet them half way. If you really want to get from A to B and have no help, then use a taxi. Think positively all the time. There is a solution to every problem if you are determined enough to seek it out. Failing sight is no excuse for being housebound.

I now use a white cane indicator when out alone, and, as the name implies, it is merely there for others to realise you have a visual problem. It works, but you will still come across the odd difficult person, like the one who told me that I had no business to be out walking the streets alone! Sorry I can't repeat my reply to that one, but even with poor vision I managed to see the guilty expression as she hurried past me! We are not disabled, just differently abled, and I find that most people with a disability pack more into their lives than an able bodied person. I know I certainly do. Interestingly I find men more considerate, understanding and willing to offer help. I wonder if visually impaired men find a reverse situation?

In a number of areas there are 'Blind Social Clubs,' although I disagree with the title. The club is certainly not 'blind' and the majority of its members are partially sighted. Despite the name, at these clubs visually impaired people can meet and chat over their various worries and problems, and even laugh at their mistakes - like ending up in the wrong loo, or on a train going in the opposite direction. One lady told me about the day she went shopping with her husband for a new dress. While she felt each garment, unknown to her he decided to wander off. Finding a dress she thought was suitable she turned, and seeing the blurred figure of a man in a similar jacket to her husband asked, 'How would you fancy me in this one?' To which the man replied, 'Lovely, but it is the first time I have been chatted up in this way!' All three managed to see the funny side of the situation. A sense of humour is essential when you are faced with such a situation. The 'Blind Club' I attend also runs a cassette library and organises various outings to theatres, river trips etc.

Any advice or tips on leisure activities?

Reading books need never be a problem for a visually impaired person. The Talking Book Service for the Blind operates an excellent service and, with over 9,000 tiles to choose from, you are spoilt for choice. The Student Cassette Library is available for those who are studying or need non-fiction books on a variety of subjects such as computing, law, history, politics etc. The RNIB also produces a large range of games for a child or adult to play with a sighted person. For example, dominoes and playing cards are available in large print and braille. There are jig-saw puzzles with raised scenes, even a bleeping ball so that a child and grandparent can play together. The Daily

Living catalogue also carries a number of products to help in the home, with labelling and writing. There are even self-threading needles or an automatic threading machine for those who enjoy sewing.

Most Resource Centres offer a range of craft materials at cost price too, as well as people who organise handicraft meetings. Check what is available in your area.

If you are arthritic too, there are many gadgets available that can help with your hobbies and leisure activities. Anglers can still enjoy fishing by using a special aid that holds the rod, and a gardener has a choice of a range of long handled tools for hoeing, weeding and picking up rubbish, as well as long-handled trowels, pruning and grass shears. However, these are often manufactured with green handles, which can become lost amongst the greenery when used by a visually impaired person. This can be rectified by wrapping a brightly coloured tape around the handle.

Any tips and advice on coping around the home?

The kitchen can be a very troublesome area for someone with failing sight and joint difficulties. A visit to your local Resource Centre can provide you with plenty of handy hints and tips. They also carry an extensive range of equipment from the RNIB catalogue and other equipment that they have found useful for people with problems. Make an appointment to go along and try them out before buying. For example there is a gadget to clip onto your cup which bleeps when the cup is almost full. Talking kitchen and bathroom scales are handy, as are the selection of braille clocks and watches or those which have large numbers or a talking mechanism.

A microwave oven is much safer to use than the conventional ones. Many Resource Centres run courses on getting the best use from it, and even have available recipes on tape.

If housework becomes difficult, invest in the services of a home help. This is money well spent, and can improve your domestic situation greatly. Most of us can cope with the general dusting and tidying, but it is the more energetic chores that sap our strength. Automatic washing machines take the hard work out of washing and can easily be operated by an arthritic or visually impaired person. Seek out new equipment on the market that will make life easier for you.

If all else fails, choose the jobs you can do and enlist help for the ones that you cannot do. Never get depressed at what you can't do. Think of all the things you can do instead, and I can guarantee that these will out-weigh the jobs that you find too difficult.

You may also have to consider changing the decor in your home to a lighter, brighter shade. Interior decorators will confirm that walls decorated with a hint of green or soft tones of pink paint give the illusion of brightness. You may find that you will need to rearrange cupboards and move shelves in order to give the best advantage of lighting. Talk to people in a similar position, and see what advice they can offer. You will always find someone who has had the same difficulty and has found a way to overcome it.

Any help or tips on coping with stress?

However well you appear to be coping with Stickler syndrome, there are bound to be times when you are under stress. Frequently it is the simple things that make us more stressful, like trying to work out the best way to get from A to B, or trying to find something that has just dropped onto the floor. I have spent hours searching for an object which, I swear, moves every time I come within an inch of it. Not being able to read a letter, a bill, or a bank statement is very frustrating too, especially when you live alone and you know that no one is going to call that day. Stress can affect anyone, at whatever stage in life, and it often leads to illness. Stress can play a part in heart disease, and doctors have established that physical breakdowns, insomnia, backache and high blood pressure can all stem from stress. Therefore, it makes sense to find ways of counteracting some of the inevitable ups and downs so that we can cope with the condition. If you follow a few basic hints life can become much less stressful.

1. Avoid any serious fatigue.
2. Keep an equal balance between rest and activity.
3. Plan a realistic programme of activities and give yourself time to achieve personal deadlines, and don't become stressed when you cannot achieve your personal goal. Allow yourself to move the goal post occasionally.

4. Try to keep some energy in reserve for that extra special outing, or that unexpected invitation.
5. Learn a relaxation technique that helps you, and practise using it when a situation produces tension.
6. If you are making your way to an appointment alone, allow yourself an extra half an hour. Then if you do end up on the wrong bus or you turn down a wrong street, you won't be too stressed, as you will have allowed yourself enough time. Try to look upon any mishaps as 'little adventures.' By doing so, you will find that the situation is less traumatic.
7. Similarly if you have been offered a lift, make sure you are ready 15 minutes before the stated time. This allows you time to collect all your belongings, and check that fires are switched off and windows locked, etc. If your lift arrives early, then again you won't be flustered if you are prepared for this.
8. Most importantly, recognise your personal limitations and have the willpower to keep within them.

If you are feeling stressed about your present situation, you may find it helps to write down all your achievements. Remember that everything you have achieved in your life that is worthwhile has been achieved despite Stickler syndrome. History is full of great people with 'something wrong' - Beethoven was deaf, yet his music is a source of pleasure to so many. Milton was blind, but he managed to write beautiful poetry, and Django Reinhardt had fingers missing, but it didn't stop him from playing the guitar. It may surprise you to know that statistics show that one person in four suffers from some sort of disability. But if you think about it, every single person suffers from some sort of incapacity. It could be that you are short and cannot reach the top shelf in the supermarket, or you may not be able to spell correctly. Perhaps cooking is your weakness or you can't put up a shelf or erect a garden shed. All these difficulties are genuine handicaps to the afflicted.

It takes real effort not to become stressed when you are 100% fit, but when you are faced with a condition like Stickler syndrome the effort needed is much greater. Think positive; you MUST make that effort. It is hard to think positively, especially when the condition is progressively restricting your movements, impairing your vision and pain is reducing you to tears, but you must NEVER give in and feel sorry for yourself.

The best way to beat stress is relaxation. There are several good tapes dealing with relaxation currently available, and I suggest that you invest in a couple. Talk to other sufferers and ask them how they cope with stress. Pick up your hobby, listen to your talking book or your favourite music, but find some way of relaxing when the tension is mounting. Personally I find writing an article or listening to music most relaxing and uplifting.

Any tips for those affected by arthritis?

Because of stiff, sore joints those affected by osteoarthritis often have difficulty in walking, bending and reaching. To overcome these problems there are many commercial products on the market, as well as aids and gadgets that help to protect the joints and prevent the development of further problems. Some people are reluctant to resort to an aid, fearing that to rely on any sort of assistance is to admit defeat or speed up the disability. Nothing could be further from the truth.

There are many aids that will help with sitting - for example the posture stool. The seat slopes forward and you sit with your weight resting on your knees and your feet tucked in underneath you. The posture stool is designed to help you to sit in a healthier position, hopefully helping you to reach the end of the day without a stiff aching back. The majority of chairs do not provide enough support for the lumber region, but there are many different types of backrests, wedges and support which help. There are even inflatable cushions which are ideal for the traveller. You may also like to consider an adjustable chair, which allows you to sit in a comfortable position, although these are expensive. Always try and sit in a chair that has arm rests so that you can rest your weight on them when sitting down or push against them when standing up. Never let your feet dangle. If a chair is too high for you, use a foot-rest, because dangling feet add to the strain on your spine. If you are seriously affected, you may like to think about buying an ejector chair which, at the touch of a lever, will help to push you up into the standing position.

If you do a lot of writing you may find a writing slope enables you to work at an angle which is better suited to your body.

Picking things up can be arduous for an arthritic sufferer, but help is at hand. There are a number of pick up sticks to make life easier, and are probably the most versatile and useful of all gadgets for the disabled. They are basically nothing more than a pair of tongs on a long handle, but can be used to close curtains, pull on socks, pick up items dropped or even lift a can or packet from a cupboard. Some have magnets on the end and others fold up so you can carry them around.

The kitchen need not present too many worries for an arthritic person, as there are many aids to help. The most useful must be the device that will open a jar. This is called a 'grip-mat' - a small non stick rubber mat that can be invaluable when opening jars, bottles or doors. There are plugs fitted with handles. There are also aids to help you lift a heavy kettle, spiked boards for peeling and chopping and cutlery with large handles.

If you find it difficult to dress yourself you will find that some clothes are unsuitable. Wear slip-on shoes and make sure that zips and buttons are large and easily accessible. Ladies may find a wrap-around skirt easy to put on. You may find it will give you some stability if you lean against a wall to dress. Roll up clothes, like jumpers so that you can put your arms through the armholes as easily as possible. If you have difficulty in balancing or pulling on trousers or tights try lying on the bed to dress. To get your trousers or tights over your feet, pull your knees up to your chest, then straighten your legs to pull your trousers or tights over your bottom. Roll your tights before placing your feet into them.

If you do have to carry shopping use a shopping trolley on wheels to relieve the strain on your back.

You may find it difficult to walk up and down stairs and you may find it helpful to ease yourself up and down on your bottom. If you are severely handicapped by the stairs investigate the possibility of installing a powered stair lift.

Can you suggest some gentle exercises?
Gentle regular exercise can help joints greatly and will allow the joint its natural range of movement, helping it to stay supple and mobile without abnormal strain. The easiest exercise, of course. is walking, but when you have a visual impairment it isn't just a simple matter of taking yourself off for a brisk walk.

Most physiotherapists can give you printed instructions on gentle exercise, but if you have a retinal problem, do please check with your ophthalmic surgeon that these exercises are appropriate.

I have outlined a few exercises, but the emphasis must be on gentle movements, slowly building up strength. Exercise regularly, preferably when you are warm from a bath or shower. If you experience giddiness at any time, STOP. These exercises are designed to help you, NOT to be used as a punishment.

GENERAL EXERCISES

Before embarking on these gentle exercises you will need an upright chair, but always remember that if you cannot make a movement, DON'T FORCE YOURSELF. Never strain yourself.

1. Sitting on the chair and keeping feet on the ground, lift up your heels, then the toes. Do this with each foot, then with both feet at the same time.
2. For neck flexibility. Let the head sag forward, but do not push, then lift it up slowly. Let your head fall gently to the side, then bring it up again. Do this for both sides.
3. Place your bottom right at the back of the chair. With your spine touching the chair back all the way up, draw yourself up - chest out, head up. Relax and repeat.
4. Sit comfortably in the chair. Drop your head forward until it touches your chest. Then gradually lean downwards towards your knees. Straighten up again, but do not unwind your head until last.

SPINE AND BACK EXERCISES

1. Stand up straight. Bend forwards towards your toes as far as you can. Then straighten up again, folding your arms across your chest, lean backwards so that you are looking towards the ceiling. Then bend forwards again. This exercise should be done as a gentle, continuous curling, starting at the base of the

spine and working upward.
2. Bend slowly sideways, running your left hand down your left thigh. Then straighten up again and do the same with the right.
3. Put your hands on your hips and, without moving your feet, rotate your spine to turn first to the right and then the to left.
4. Lie as flat as possible on a bed, and press the head and shoulders hard back into the bed. Relax and repeat.
5. Using your tummy muscles, lift the head up to look at the feet.
6. Sitting in an upright chair, lean backwards arching your back whilst taking a deep breath in. Relax and breathe out. Repeat.
7. Sit up straight in a chair and twist the body round to look behind, keeping your bottom squarely on the chair. Repeat the exercise turning the other way.
8. Lean forward to put the head on the knees, straighten to the upright position slowly.

EXERCISES FOR THE FEET AND ANKLES

1. Sit with legs crossed and pull feet up and down from the ankle. When pushing down point the toes hard towards the floor. Repeat with the other foot.
2. Circle the foot round from the ankle drawing a large circle in the air with the big toe. Repeat with the other foot.
3. Press the toes flat against the floor and, keeping them straight, raise the ball of the foot off the ground to make a bridge. This

is a very important exercise to re-train the small 'sling' muscles supporting the arches of the foot. Repeat with the other foot.

KNEES

1. Lie on your back with your knees outstretched. Slowly bend up one knee as far as it will go, then stretch the leg out straight again. Then do the same with your other leg.
2. Lie straight with your feet pointing upwards. Slowly lift one leg - not very high, but just enough so that it is not touching the bed. Keeping your knee straight and your thigh muscles braced, lower it again slowly until the calf touches the bed and then relax. Repeat the exercise with each leg in turn.

SHOULDERS

1. Sit on an upright dining chair. Let one arm hang down by the side and swing it forwards and backwards in a pendular movement. Repeat with the other arm.
2. With the arm hanging as before, swing it away from the side.
3. Support the hand and wrist with your other hand, raise the elbow away from the side.
4. Lift and circle the shoulders, first one way and then the other, trying each time for the maximum mobility.

    All these exercises should be done for short periods, with a rest between.

USEFUL ORGANISATIONS AND ADDRESSES

LOOK - National Federation of Families with Visually Impaired Children - Queen Alexandra College, 49 Court Oak Road, Birmingham, B17 0TG Tel: 0121-428-5038.

Look is the only national organisation that concentrates on providing practical help and support for families with visually impaired children. They have local groups throughout the UK and can provide guidance concerning the real meaning behind the complex medical terms used by doctors. The organisation will advise parents on their child's entitlement to social security and welfare benefits and offer practical information and advice on toys and games that are available to stimulate a visually impaired child. They will explain what is meant by 'statementing', and offer information on the local and national educational choices.

STICKLER SYNDROME SUPPORT GROUP - Mrs Wendy Hughes, 27 Braycourt Avenue, Walton on Thames, Surrey, KT12 2AZ Tel: 01932 229421.

The Stickler Syndrome Support Group was set up to help those affected and their families to cope with the day to day management of the condition. The group can provide timely information about the disorder to patients, their families and the medical profession. It can help by putting families in touch with others who have similar difficulties through their parents network system, and offers mutual support and aims to share information. The group also operates a Youngster Network for teenagers and young adults to link up with others to support each other and share ideas. Publications available include a quarterly newsletter and factfiles on various aspects of the condition.

CONTACT-A-FAMILY - 170 Tottenham Court Road, London, W1P OHA Tel: 0171-383-3555.

This is an organisation offering advice and information to parents with children suffering from a rare syndrome. They also publish a directory entitled the *Contact a Family Directory of Specific Conditions and Rare Syndromes in Children.* This includes information on over 200 conditions from Addison's Disease to Wolf-Hirschhorn syndrome and gives details of all UK family support networks.

CLAPA - The Cleft Lip and Palate Association. National Secretary, Mrs Cy Thirlaway, 1 Eastwood Gardens, Kenton, Newcastle-upon-Tyne NE3 3DG. Tel: 0191-285-9396.

CLAPA offers support, especially to parents of the new born child. The Group comprises of parents, nurses, and professionals from a variety of disciplines: Maxillofacial surgeons, dental specialists, psychologists, speech therapists, and social workers: all linked by experience or vocation to an understanding of the needs and treatment of those with cleft lip or cleft palate. They are jointly concerned to help such individuals to look better, speak better and adjust better.

IN TOUCH - Mrs Ann Worthington MBE, 10 Norman Road, Sale, Cheshire, M33 3DF Tel: 061-905-2440.

Information and contacts for parents of children with special needs

GIG - Genetic Interest Group - Farringdon Point, 29-35 Farringdon Road, London, EC1M 3JB Tel: 0171-430-0092

GIG is the umbrella group of voluntary organisations concerned with Genetic Disorders, working to benefit all people affected by genetic disorders.

THE LADY HOARE TRUST - for physically disabled children, 4th Floor, Mitre House, 44-46 Fleet Street, London, EC4Y 1BN Tel: 0171-583-1951.

The Trust can offer practical and financial help to children up to the age of 18 who are physically disabled by arthritis or limb problems.

RNIB - Royal National Institute For the Blind - PO Box 173, Peterborough, Cambs PE2 OWS. Direct line to customer services 0345-023153.

A call to this number is charged at a local rate, and will produce an information pack on all facilities available.

PARTIALLY SIGHTED SOCIETY - Queen's Road Doncaster DN1 2NX Tel: 01302-323132.

The society was founded in 1973 and is now a registered charity with a national office and over twenty local self-help branches. It offers advice on all aspects of living and working with a visual loss and can offer a range of equipment.

MARFAN ASSOCIATION SUPPORT GROUP - Mrs D Rust, 6 Queen's Road, Farnborough, Hants, GU14 6DH
Tel: 01252-547441

The Association advises individuals and their families who are affected by this inherited disorder.

TADPOLES DEVELOPMENTAL GLAUCOMA SUPPORT GROUP - c\o Mrs Jackie Drewett, 65 Bush Barns, West Cheshunt, Hertfordshire, EN7 6ED.

Supporting parents of babies and young children with glaucoma

SENSE - THE NATIONAL DEAFBLIND AND RUBELLA ASSOCIATION - 11-13 Clifton Terrace, Finsbury Park, London, N4 3SR Tel: 0171-272-7774.

Although a child may not be deaf and blind, this organisation can help families with multi-disabilities.

TALKING BOOK SERVICE - Mount Pleasant, Wembley Middlesex, HAO 1RR Tel: 0181-903-666.

CALIBRE - Aylesbury, Buckinghamshire, HP22 5XQ
Tel: 01296-432339.

This is a lending library of recorded books on standard cassette. It is available to anyone who cannot read ordinary print, and membership is on production of a doctor's certificate. Those who are registered need only send a photocopy of their registration certificate.

THE TALKING NEWSPAPER ASSOCIATION - 90 High Street, Heathfield, East Sussex, TN21 8JD Tel: 01435-866102.

The Association produces over 90 weekly, monthly and quarterly publications on standard cassette. £10 per year entitles you to receive as many titles as you wish.

INTERNATIONAL GLAUCOMA ASSOCIATION - Kings College Hospital, Denmark Hill, London, SE5 9RS Tel: 0171-737-3265

RESOURCE CENTRES

There are many resource centres throughout Britain which are run by the Social Service Department of local councils, Blind Associations and others. It is not practical to list these here and if you wish to avail yourself of their facilities your social workers or doctor should be able to help. You can also try the local library or look them up in the telephone directory.

SOME HELPFUL AIDS

THE HABERMAN FEEDER Bottle - Athrodax Surgical Limited, Great Western Court, Ashburton, Ross on Wye, HR9 7XP Tel: 01989-566669

MEAD JOHNSON VERY SOFT BOTTLE, CHICCO WIDE NECKED BOTTLE AND ROSTI SOFT BOTTLE - All these bottles and other feeding equipment are available from CLAPA'S

Feeding Equipment Co-Ordinator: Jan Robertson, 6 Blenheim Close, Danbury, Essex CM3 4NE. Tel: 01245-225657 (24 hour answerphone)

THE EEZEE READER - The Force Ten Co Limited, 183 Boundary Road, Woking, Surrey, GU21 5BU.

GLOSSARY OF TERMS

ALLELE - Alternative forms of a gene found at the same locus on homologous chromosomes.

ARTHROPATHY - Any disease or disorder involving a joint.

AUDIOGRAM - the graphic record of a hearing test carried out on a audiometer.

AUTOSOME - A non sex determining chromosome - any chromosome other than the X and Y chromosome.

CONGENITAL - Existing at birth.

COXA VALGA - Deformity of the hip joint in which the angle made by the neck and shaft of the femur is greater than normal.

D.N.A. - Deoxyribonucleic acid - the genetic material of nearly all living organisms which controls heredity, and is located in the cell nucleus. DNA is a nucleic acid composed of two strands made up of units called nucleotide. The two strands are wound around each other into a double helix and linked together by hydrogen bonds between the bases of the nucleotide. The genetic information of the DNA is contained in the sequence of bases along the molecule. Changes in the DNA cause mutations. The DNA molecule can make exact copies of itself by the process of replication, thereby passing on the genetic information to the daughter cells when the cell divides.

FIBROSITIS - Inflammation of fibrous connective tissue, especially an acute inflammation of back muscles and their sheaths, causing pain and stiffness.

GLAUCOMA - A condition in which loss of vision occurs because of an abnormally high pressure in the eye. This may occur when other ocular disease impairs the normal circulation of the aqueous humour and causes the intra-ocular pressure to rise.

KYPHOSIS - Hump back - Angular deformity of the spine.

LESIONS - Tissue that is impaired as a result of damage by disease or wounding.

MALOCCLUSION - Bad contact between the chewing surfaces of the upper and lower teeth.

MANDIBULAR - Relating to the lower jaw.

MAXILLARY - Relating to the upper jaw.

MICROGNATHIA - Abnormal smallness of the jaws, especially the lower jaw.

MUTATION - A change in the genetic material of a cell. All mutations are rare events and may occur spontaneously or be caused by external agents.

MYOPIA - shortsightedness (nearsightedness).

NYSTAGMUS - Rapid involuntary movement of the eyes that may be from side to side, up and down, or rotatory, and may be associated with poor vision.

OPHTHALMOLOGIST - a doctor who specialises in the diagnosis and treatment of eye diseases.

OTITIS MEDIA - or glue ear. This occurs when the tube linking the middle ear to the back of the nose becomes blocked, and a jelly-like fluid, naturally secreted by the ear, is unable to drain away. The mucus becomes thicker, filling the middle-ear and reducing hearing to a muffled roar.

PECTUS - Chest or thorax

PROBAND OR PROPOSITUS - The first individual studied in an investigation of several related patients with an inherited or familial disorder.

PROGNOSIS - An assessment for the future

PROPHYLAXIS - Any means taken to prevent a disease.

RHEUMATOLOGIST - a doctor who specialises in the diagnosis and management of joint disease.

SCOLIOSIS - Lateral curvature of the spine

STRABISMUS - Squint, when the eye diverts.

SYNDROME - a collection of signs and symptoms that form a distinct picture of a particular disorder.

TALIPES ENQIUNOVARUS - Club foot with the heel lifted from the ground.

READING LIST

1. **ARE YOU BLIND?** by Lilli Nielson, published by Sikon.
   A book designed for parents and professionals on coping with visually impaired children.

2. **A SENSORY CURRICULUM FOR SPECIAL PEOPLE** by Flo Longhon, published Human Horizon Series 1988 Souvenir Press.
   A source book of ideas to stimulate all the child's senses.

3. **UNDERSTANDING THE DEAF/BLIND CHILD** by Peggy Freeman, published by Wm Heinemann Medical Books Limited 1975.

4. **MOBILITY TRAINING FOR VISUALLY HANDICAPPED PEOPLE** by Alan Dodds, published Croom Helm 1988.

5. **KITCHEN SENSE FOR DISABLED OR ELDERLY PEOPLE,** published for Disabled Living Foundation by Wm Heinemann Medical Books Limited 1975.
   Easy recipes and helpful hints for the visually impaired.

6. **EASY TO MAKE TOYS FOR YOUR HANDICAPPED CHILD** by Don Caston published Human Horizons Series 1983 Souvenir Press Ltd.

7   **IN TOUCH HANDBOOK** - by BBC, available from BBC Support Services, PO BOX 7, London, W3 6XJ.
This handbook has become the standard reference book for anyone concerned with visually impaired people. A valuable guide to aids and services available.

8   **DISABILITY RIGHTS HANDBOOK** Available from Disability Alliance. ERA, Universal House, 88-94 Wentworth Street, London E1 7SA.
Best guide available on the benefits system.

9. **50 POPULAR TOYS FOR BLIND AND PARTIALLY SIGHTED CHILDREN** - a booklet produced by the RNIB. Tel 01345 023153 for a copy.

A list of other useful books can be obtained from: RNIB Reference Library, 224 Great Portland Street London W1N 6AA Tel: 0171-388-1266

LIST OF MEDICAL REFERENCES

1. Hereditary Progressive Arthro-ophthalmopathy, by Stickler, Belau, Farrell, Pugh, Steinberg and Ward. Mayo Clinic Proceedings Vol 40 June 1965 pages 433-455.
2. Hereditary Progressive Arthro-ophthalmopathy. Additional Observations on Vertebral abnormalities. A hearing defect, and a report of a similar case, by Stickler and Pugh. Mayo Clinic Proceedings Vol 42 August 1967, page 495-500.
3. Ocular Anomalies in Malformation Syndromes, John M Opitz MD, Trans American Acad Ophthal. and Otol. Vol 76 1972, pages 1193-1202.
4. The Stickler Syndrome, Opitz,France, Herrmann, Spranger, New England Journal of Med. Vol 286 pages 546-547.
5. Stickler Syndrome in a Pedigree of Pierre Robin Syndrome. Schreiner, McAlister, Marshall, Shearer. Am. J. Dis. Child. Vol 126 July 1973, pages 86-90.
6. The Stickler Syndrome in a family with the Pierre Robin Syndrome and Severe Myopia. Gillian Turner. Australiam Paediatric Journal 1974 pages 103-108.
7. Stickler Syndrome (Hereditary Progressive Arthro-

ophthalmopathy). Popkin, Polimeno. Canadian Medical Association Journal Nov 16 1974 Vol 111 (10). pages 1071-1076.

8. The Stickler Syndrome (Hereditary Artho-ophthalmopathy). Herrmann, France, Spranger, Opitz and Wiffler. Birth Defects. 1975 Vol X1 no 2.

9. Stickler Syndrome by I K Temple, Journal of Medical Genetics Feb, 1989 Vol 26 (2) pages 119-126.

10. The Stickler Syndrome is closely linked to COL2A1, the structural gene of type 11 collagen, by Fransomano, Liberfarb, Hirose, Manmenee. Streeten. Meyers, Pyeritz. Pathol-Immunopathol - Res 1988 Vol 7 (1-2) pages 104-106.

11. Stickler Syndrome: A study of 12 Families, by A Spallone. British Journal of Ophthalmol July 1987 Vol 71 (7) Pages 504-509.

12. Management of Retinal Detachment in the Wagner-Stickler Syndrome, by Billington, Leaver, McLoed. Transworld Ophthalmol Society U.K. 1965 Col 104, Pages 675-679.

13. Stickler Syndrome and Neovascular Glaucoma, by Young, Hitchings, Sehmi, Bird. British Journal of Ophthalmol Dec 1978 Vol 63, pages 826-831.

14. The Stickler Syndrome presenting as a dominantly inherited cleft palate and blindness, by Hall, Herrod. Journal Medical Genetics Dec 1975 Vol 12 (4) pages 390-400.

15. Congenital Myopia and retinal detachment. by J.D Scott Trans Ophthalmol Soc UK, 1980, 100 pages 69-71.
16. Giant Tear of the Retina by J. D. Scott. Trans Ophthalmol Soc UK 1975, 95 pages 142-4.
17. Stickler Syndrome: Correlation Between Vitreoretinal Phenotypes and Linkage to COL2A1. Snead, Payne, Barton, Yates, Al-Imera, Pope and Scott.

    Royal College of Ophthalmologists Eye (1994) 8, 609-614.

BIBLIOGRAPHY

1. Elements of Medical Genetics by Emery and Mueller, Pub. Churchill Livinstone.
2. Basic Biochemistry by Edelman and Chapman, Pub. Wm Heinemann.
3. The Genetic Jigsaw: The story of the New Genetics, by Robin McKie, pub. Oxford University Press 1988.
4. Dictionary of Nature by David Burnie, Pub, Dorling Kindersley 1994.

ABOUT THE AUTHOR

Wendy Hughes was born in South Wales and now lives in Walton on Thames Surrey with her husband and two grown up sons. She turned to writing as an outlet for her frustrations when ill health and poor vision forced her to give up work. During this period her writing proved most therapeutic and helped her to cope with many sight-saving operations. In 1988 she was finally diagnosed as suffering from Stickler Syndrome, and this diagnosis coupled with the acceptance of her first article enabled her to come to terms with her difficulties and to take up a new career as a writer. Since that first acceptance she has had over 600 articles published, including several on Stickler Syndrome. She writes regularly for several magazines including Ninnau, an American\Welsh newspaper for ex-patriots, Funeral Service Journal, On The Road, and Country Quest.

STICKLER - THE ELUSIVE SYNDROME is her seventh book, and two more are planned for publication in 1996. After years of being misdiagnosed and misunderstood she vowed that she would help others by raising awareness of the condition, founding the Stickler Syndrome Support Group and writing this book.

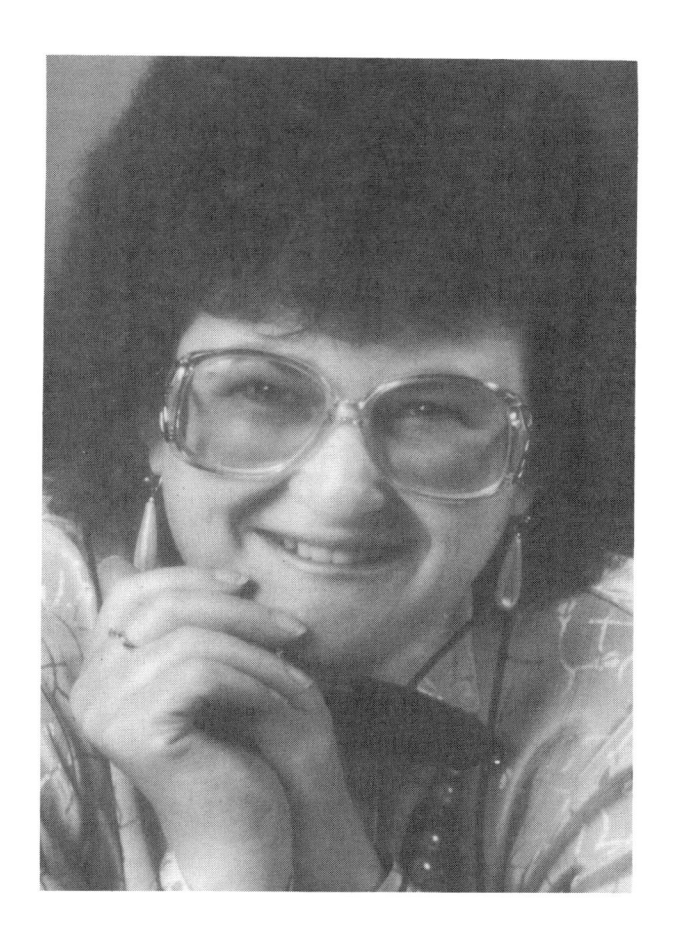

The Author

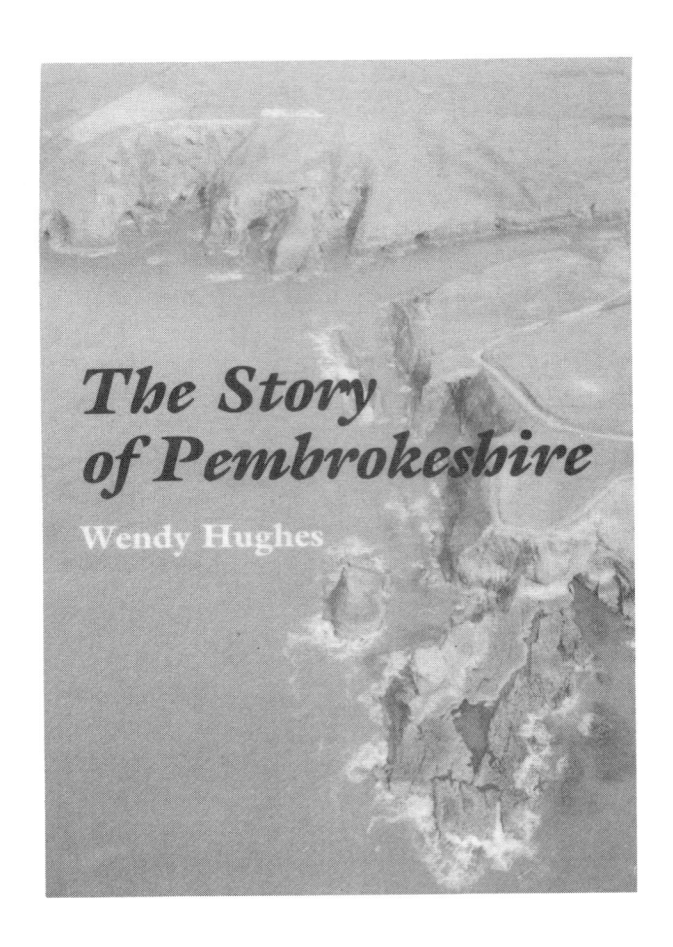

The Story of Pembrokeshire *100pp. £3.00. 0-86381-253-8.
Black & white illustrations.*
Pembrokeshire is an area that rose from the sea over
thousand million years, and has since played host to paga
warriors, Celtic fort-builders, Welsh princes, swashbucklin
pirates, Manx shearwaters, and the Grey Atlantic seal.
Wendy Hughes

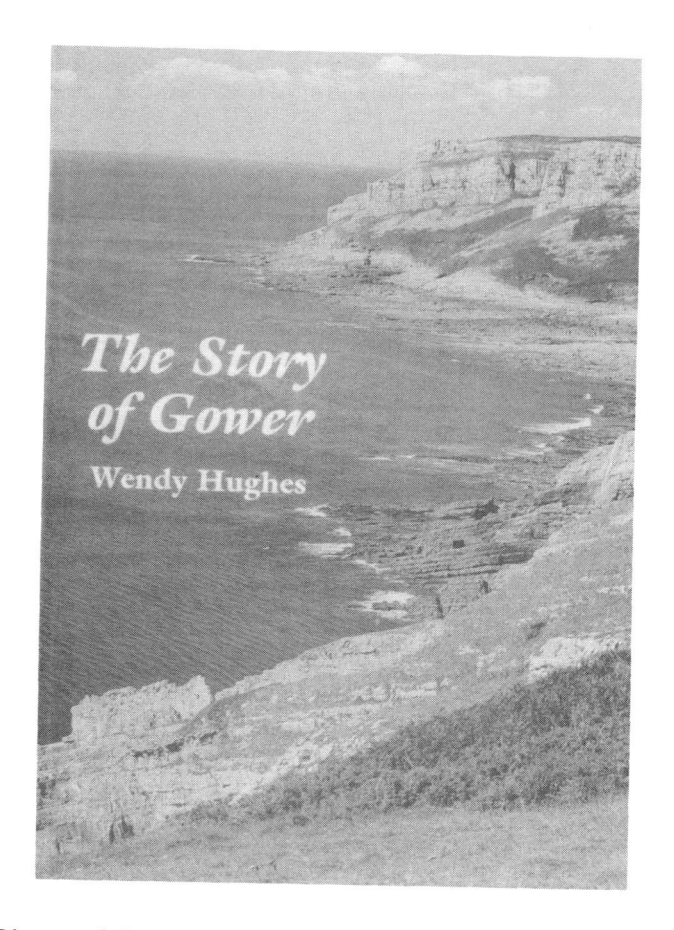

The Story of Gower 88pp. £2.75. 0-86381-217-1.
Many illustrations.
Wendy Hughes' *Story of Gower*, takes the reader from the cave dwellers icy existence to modern day Gower, drawing on a richly woven pageant of history, legends and notorious characters, that will hold the readers attention until the last page is turned.
Wendy Hughes

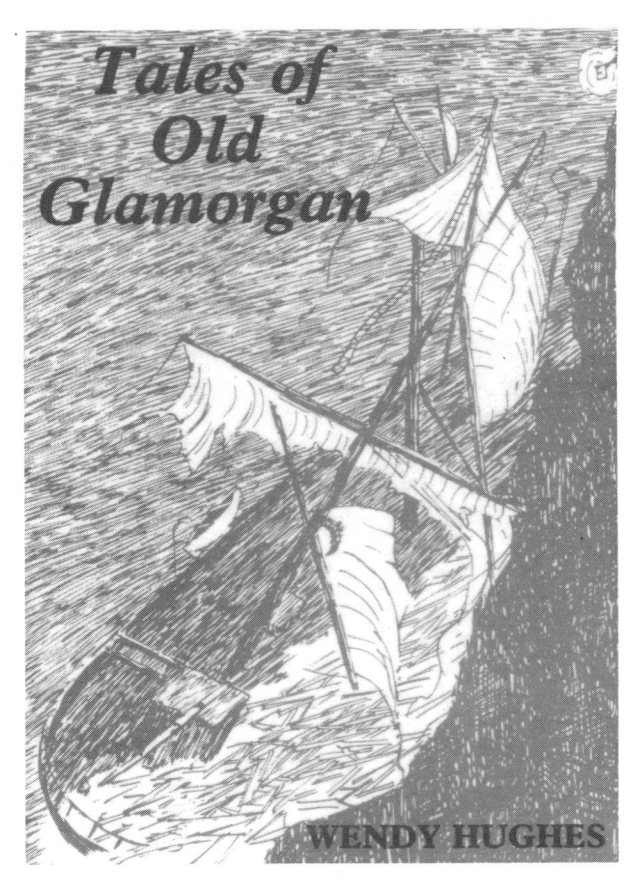

Tales of Old Glamorgan *132pp. £4.25. 0-86381-287-2.*
Black & white illustrations.
The art of story telling is deeply rooted in Welsh tradition. In this book, Wendy Hughes captivates the very essence of this culture and brings alive the tales which lie at the heart of the county of Glamorgan — legends, fables of fairies and magic, foxes and snakes, myths to enchant as well as stories of devils, witches and ghosts.
Wendy Hughes